The Gentle Birth Method

The Month-by-Month Jeyarani Way Programme

Dr Gowri Motha and Karen Swan MacLeod

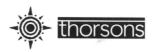
thorsons

Thorsons
An Imprint of HarperCollins*Publishers*
77–85 Fulham Palace Road,
Hammersmith, London W6 8JB

The website address is:
www.thorsonselement.com

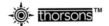

and *Thorsons* are trademarks of
HarperCollins*Publishers* Ltd

First published by Thorsons 2004

13

A catalogue record of this book
is available from the British Library

ISBN-13   978-0-00-717684-7
ISBN-10   0-00-717684-8

Printed and bound in Great Britain by
Martins the Printers, Berwick upon Tweed

Contents

Acknowledgements

DR GOWRI MOTHA

I would like to thank the following people:

Alison Maclaine – my friend and creative editor. Over the last 10 years Ali has been patiently collating my teaching material and research findings. She said that all this material could be a book one day and, by formalizing The Jeyarani Way Gentle Birth Method, laid the foundation for this book. Her gift of patience and her tolerance of my timetable and out of hours working deserves great acknowledgement. Ali I honour the hard work and the selfless support that you have given me all these years. A big thank you also to Geraldine for the hours of work that you have selflessly given to our work. Thank you Fergus for your advice and support. Thank you 'Maclaines' – you are precious.

Karen Swan MacLeod – for your love and insight into the Jeyarani Way Gentle Birth Method, and for manifesting this book. Without your enthusiasm this book would have never come into being. My heartfelt thanks to you Karen, and to Anders your special husband, and of course Ollie and the darling new baby on the way.

Kasia Ogonowska – who has helped me to establish the Jeyarani Gentle Birth clinic at Viveka at St John's Wood. Kasia's excellence as a Jeyarani Way birth therapist is based on her empathy for our mothers and in her ability to communicate our message of gentle birthing. Her dedication to the details of our practice has contributed greatly to its success. Kasia you have been a strength to me in countless ways.

Marion Mackay – when we met on a reflexology course that I was teaching 10 years ago, I knew that we were meant to meet. She reminded me that I was previously her NHS doctor for three of her eight babies! Marion was the first therapist that I trained and I wanted her innate wisdom and ability to give birth easily to inspire all the mothers on my programme. I have learnt much from her. Thank you for being my first student and a champion of my methods. Your healing hands have helped hundreds of mothers and I look forward to a long working life together.

Debbie Linger – the kindest person I know, started off as one of my mothers in 1994, and now shares my passion for helping other mothers. Debbie is distinguished by her ability to exhibit extreme sensitivity and love to all she comes in contact with. She is closely involved with her three children's education and development and I wonder where she gets all her energy. Debbie has proved to be an excellent practitioner and I am confident she will continue to develop and carry on the Jeyarani Way in order to benefit the next few generations.

Sherine Lovegrove – thank you for inspiring me to formalize and teach the Creative Healing and the birth therapist course. Sherine is a midwife, hypnotherapist and reflexologist, and a powerful member of our team. She also co-teaches the courses.

A big thank you also to all those practitioners who have given their time generously to the development of the Jeyarani Way Gentle Birth Method – Viola Martens, Helen Dennis, Chika Nagasu (Tokyo), Fiona Meeks, Heather Guerrini, Barbara Stanhope-Williams, Judith Davies and Marysia Kelly.

Lynne Howard – for joining my circle of close friends and for your generous contributions on homoeopathy, which have been included in this book.

Dr Palitha Serasinghe – for his expert advice on Ayurveda.

Susanna Hall – for her insight into the Bowen technique and also for teaching me the method.

Agnes Soden – my friend and spiritual mother in London. Apart from being the only living saint that I know, Agnes has encouraged me and kept me focused on my work. Her prayers, scones and cups of tea have kept me going for 23 years in London.

Riet Warmerdam – who has helped me in so many ways to keep up my morale. She and late husband Piet generously included me in their intimate circle of family and friends and gave me a family in London.

Patricia and John Bradley – my Creative Healing teachers and friends from California. As visionaries for the Creative Healing method, they have given their rich retirement years to teaching it worldwide. Thank you both for being my mentors and for your love. I love you both.

Yehudi Gordon – my friend and colleague who created Viveka, a clinic dedicated to integrating complementary medicine into Obs/Gyn medicine. Yehudi has promoted The Jeyarani Way Gentle Birth Method and this has enabled us to work together with several mothers. Working alongside Yehudi at Viveka has been a nurturing experience for my practitioners and me. Thank you Yehudi.

Laurence Wood (obstetric consultant) – for his ongoing interest in my work and for inviting me on several occasions to talk about my work.

Michel Odent – for inspiring me since the early days of the Jeyarani centre 1987. Thank you for your friendship and your weekly presence at our singing groups for pregnant mothers. We all love you.

I thank my late mother Jeyarani Motha for her sensitive observations on life, which have imprinted on me deeply. I honour her memory by giving her name to The Jeyarani Way Gentle Birth Method. I thank my late father Benedict Motha, whose work as a doctor fascinated me as a child. His enormous love for the art of medicine created a curiosity in me that made me study medicine just to find out what it was that he loved so much! Apart from the agony of being a medical student, medicine has given me great opportunities and wonderful moments of excitement. I thank my family in India who generously let me go to 'find myself' in the West. What a ride it has been!

I thank God for the Divine protection that my mothers and I have received.

I thank all my teachers, friends and colleagues and mothers too numerous to name, for their trust, love and enthusiasm for life. I am also grateful for all my life experiences, the good times and the difficult times, because without them both one cannot measure the other. I am also grateful for the opportunity to work in London – it has allowed me to develop both mentally and spiritually.

KAREN SWAN MACLEOD
I would like to firstly thank my husband, Anders, for his constant support, strong love and beautiful babies; my parents for their unstinting love, devotion and presence in our lives; my beloved son Oliver, who inspired me to become involved in this project, and who underpins everything I do. And finally, I must thank Gowri, for giving us the greatest start on the road to being a happy family together.

Preface

by Elle Macpherson

I first met Gowri when I was pregnant with my second son. My first labour had been quite long and although I knew this one was likely to be shorter, I wanted, if not a guarantee to a pain-free, 20-minute birth, at least the inside track to a shortcut. Who wouldn't? We all want to hurry up and meet our babies, after all.

Gowri explained to me quite early on in my pregnancy that, with guided preparations, I could have as natural – and short – a birth as nature intended for me, so I was more than happy to put in the groundwork. Daily exercise and a healthy diet are a part of my lifestyle anyway, but with international travel as a regular feature in my schedule, it was really important for me to feel rooted during my pregnancy. I particularly found the visualisations and hypnotic birth rehearsals allowed me to 'nest' and concentrate on the baby, regardless of whether I was 35,000 feet in the air, or two days' travel away from home.

And it worked for me! I had an incredibly positive, emotional, and nurturing waterbirth. I delivered my son on my due date after a relatively short four-hour labour. It was the most amazing experience I've ever had, and thanks to Gowri's preparation I was able to cope with the pain and be 100 per cent present without drugs for the incredible moment of his birth. To add to my joy I did not tear or need to have an episiotomy.

Now I send all my girlfriends to Gowri's clinic as soon as they tell me they're expecting. She's been one of my best-kept secrets – until now.

Foreword

by Dr Yehudi Gordon

It is a great pleasure to write the foreword for Gowri Motha's book on Gentle Birth. As a fellow obstetrician with a similar passion for natural, active and water births, I believe that Gowri's philosophy, approach and incredible enthusiasm are an inspiration and great help for women. I can vouch through experience that women who have met and worked with Gowri and her team are far more likely to have a gentle, natural birth.

Gowri is a fully trained obstetrician and gynaecologist. Gowri was born in Sri Lanka and completed her training in India, so the principles and practices of Ayurveda are second nature to her. In her birth preparation work she teams up with a group of like-minded women. Gowri is, above all, a team player, with each pregnant woman and her baby taking centre stage.

Gowri calls her birth preparation 'Jeyarani'. On a foundation of Ayurveda she combines aspects from a number of disciplines, including nutrition and complementary therapies, such as reflexology, massage, healing, Bowen, Reiki and Cranio-sacral therapy. The accent is on helping women feel profoundly in touch with their bodies and their babies and building their confidence in their natural ability to give birth.

The term 'midwife' means, literally, 'with woman' and conveys a role of shared wisdom and loving support. Gowri's team of therapists helps a pregnant mother feel loved, valued, secure and held at a number of levels. Physically, each woman is encouraged to release strain and tension throughout her body, with particular focus on the birthing areas and on the breath. Emotionally, she is welcomed, her feelings are acknowledged and valued, and her confidence is boosted: the Jeyarani technique creates a space that allows each woman to be who she is and access her own very special power to nurture herself and her baby, and prepare for birth. Midwives work from the outside, but the Jeyarani preparation programme encourages the woman's internal midwife and mothering to blossom.

Visualization plays an important role. Each woman is guided to visualize her power as a woman, the power of her contractions and most importantly the ability of her body to open and give birth. This builds self-confidence and harmonizes body, mind and spirit. The experience of preparation is a source of joy: apprehension and fear diminish and women tend to feel wholly in touch with themselves. Women are also encouraged to eat well, exercise and stretch with Yoga. Gowri also teaches gentle self-massage of the vagina and perineum, which brings women in touch with this important birth area and prepares it for opening and stretching at birth, acting as a type of bio-feedback to release tension.

The Jeyarani programme does not focus exclusively on pregnancy and birth: Gowri also encourages women to consider their transition to motherhood and look ahead to bonding with their babies, and adjusting to the birth of a new family.

The stories in this book speak for themselves and are a testament to the Jeyarani Birth Preparation method, but above all to Gowri and her team, who encourage pregnant women to tune into, believe and exercise their power. Working with Gowri does not automatically guarantee a natural birth, as there are many different variables that affect each baby's unique entry to the world. It does however, make it much more likely. It is a privilege to attend the labours of women who have been assisted by Gowri, and to celebrate the births of their babies who have been welcomed and lovingly nurtured throughout pregnancy.

Introduction

I have always been bemused by the fact that, as pregnant women, we spend longer preparing the nursery for the baby, than our bodies. We sigh over wallpaper swatches, pore over name books and coo over cots without once thinking about conditioning ourselves for birth. Perhaps the inevitability of it just leaves us wanting to bury our heads in the sand, anxiously awaiting those first rumbling contractions, or maybe the thought of it is just too frightening to contemplate. After all, birth is packaged to us as a traumatic, painful and undignified rite of passage that nearly every woman – sooner or later – must go through. Who would want to dwell on that? And yet, we must. The statistics bear out these preconceived notions of what birth must be like: a recent survey reported that over 80 per cent of women were frightened during labour and 53 per cent found giving birth 'far more shocking' than they thought it would be. It's a two-fold problem. On the one hand, some women's expectations are not being managed, so the birthing experience is a raw shock for them; on the other, there are those women who are going into labour fully expecting it to be horrendous, and so it is. A big part of this latter problem is that the vast majority of young women who are now at childbearing age have grown up with the received wisdom that this is how birth is. But it isn't what I grew up with. Born in Sri Lanka and educated in India, my notion of childbirth was rooted in a far simpler reality – that it is natural, quick and even reasonably gentle. Please don't misread 'gentle' for 'painless', it isn't and I don't want to imply that at all. But it is manageable and let's not forget that as a physical function that has been honed over centuries, childbirth is actually what our bodies are best at.

I only met this negative attitude to birth when I came to England and was struck by the irony that the sophisticated technology that has made childbirth safer for women than ever before has also made it harder. Over-stretched doctors, fearful of complications and litigation, are too quick to intervene at the first sign of difficulty, steadily undermining the fact that childbirth is a naturally occurring event that women are fully capable of achieving.

I should know – I was one of those doctors. As an obstetrician working at various hospitals around London, I delivered hundreds of babies. Unfortunately, most of the mothers were rigid with fear, in poor physical condition and emotionally out of control. By the time I saw them, the best I could do was administer an epidural and apply the forceps. The medical community's attitude towards childbirth was, and is, of crisis management, of dealing with the complications the pregnant mothers were exhibiting once in labour. Very little thought was given to stopping the problems before they started, of getting to the root of the problem. So I began to wonder – could the quality of a mother's pregnancy determine her labour experience? If she primed herself with physical stamina and mental resilience, could she condition herself for birth, like an athlete training for a race?

That was 15 years ago and today I have refined my results into a concise birth preparation programme that will hone your body and mind for the birthing process. The programme works on three levels. The first tackles your physical condition, aiming to detoxify and decongest your body through a wholefood diet, physical treatments and daily exercise. The idea is to purify your body so that there is no residual muscle tension, water retention or joint stiffness to impede the pelvic opening and loosening that is a necessary precursor for a gentle birth.

The second level addresses your mental attitude and any resistance you may have towards pregnancy – even if the baby was planned – or any fears about the birth. To do this, we move through carefully conceived visualization and self-hypnosis techniques that re-evaluate your feelings, develop your mental strength and give you the confidence to manage your contractions and remain in control of your labour. And finally, we engage on an emotional level – extending a loving welcome to your unborn baby and learning how to bond with your baby in the womb.

The fact that this programme is holistic and yet underpinned by sound medical judgement and experience means that The Gentle Birth Method is a unique approach to pregnancy and birth. However, if I had to stipulate the fundamental difference between this book and many other pregnancy guides, it is that this is a comprehensive programme for you to follow every day of your pregnancy. It isn't a reference guide to pick up as and when you have a query, or want a homoeopathic remedy to an ailment. Nor is it a theoretical textbook about pregnancy and childbirth. This book goes further than any other by giving you a framework that shows you how to 'be' pregnant. The general attitude towards pregnancy is that it is a passive state of being, something that 'happens' to you for nine months. But I firmly believe pregnancy is an interactive, dynamic condition that you can nurture and mould to your own expectations. So keep this book in your handbag, in your desk at work, or on your bedside table – you're going to find it an invaluable aid.

The Gentle Birth Method is for all mothers, whatever their age, culture, religion, or social status. And it isn't just for the first-time mother either. In fact, in many ways, it is more relevant to those women who have already had a pregnancy or birth experience. If you have had a traumatic first birth and are terrified of repeating the whole experience – and a shocking amount of women are – this book is for you. If you have tragically suffered a miscarriage or stillbirth, then this programme can help you. Of course, it cannot offer cures to the specific clinical conditions that may have undermined the viability of your previous pregnancy, nor can it change your past. But, by giving you a specific weekly framework within which to operate, you can concentrate on nurturing this baby. The difference this time around is that you are now making yourself ready for the birthing experience.

By the time you read the last page of this book, birth won't be able to frighten, overwhelm or surprise you. You will know how to reduce the amount of pain you feel, and the clever little shortcuts to full cervical dilatation. You will know not only what is happening to your body during childbirth, but also your baby's. And whilst it's doing all this, The Gentle Birth Method will cosset you, restore your faith and return birth to you as a joyous, happy event that is neither feared, nor needs to be interfered with.

More than 1200 mothers have followed the Gentle Birth programme and our results consistently show that we have improved birth for women and their babies. Our figures for total time spent in labour, intervention (i.e. epidurals, ventouse, forceps), episiotomies and Caesarean sections dramatically undercut the national averages and are clear proof that there is another way for women. But numbers aren't the motivation for The Gentle Birth Method. Motherhood is the greatest gift and it deserves a happy beginning. It is my hope that this programme will help you celebrate pregnancy as one of the most precious chapters in your life, and equip you with the potential for a birth that is a calm, intimate and bonding experience for both you and your baby.

DR GOWRI MOTHA

SECTION A

Preparing for Birth

Physical Preparation

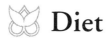 **Diet**

If you imagine that pregnancy means waddling, puffing up stairs and being the size of a house, then you're going to be pleased you bought this book. Because if there's one thing that characterizes absolutely all the mothers who follow my programme, it's this – they're light on their feet.

At nine months, when most expectant mothers can't get their shoes on, mine have a spring in their step. When most can't get off the sofa, mine go off on a two-mile walk – they've got energy, confidence and excitement, and the only water they retain is kept in a bottle in their handbags.

You've heard of those women who are back in their pre-pregnancy clothes two weeks after giving birth – well, you could be one of them. I'm not advocating no weight gain during pregnancy by any means – in fact it's crucial that mothers lay down some fat – but I do believe that mothers should control their weight gain in order to modulate the size of their baby. Babies are definitely bigger when the mother is overweight and both factors – big babies and overweight mummies – lead to a higher incidence of complicated births. My studies show that an optimum-sized baby for a mother of average build leads to a gentler birth – and less incidence of post-natal depression, because the mother doesn't have to add getting her figure back to her 'To Do' list.

How can this sort of pregnancy be yours? Well, in the first instance, by following a simple diet. But before you gasp with horror at the thought of expectant mothers on diets, this is absolutely not about losing weight, deprivation or hunger. Yes, it does involve excluding certain foods – I ask all my mothers to cut out wheat, refined carbohydrates (puddings, chocolate, bread, biscuits and so on) and, in the last month, gluten – but here's why.

When I was working as an obstetrician in an NHS hospital, the same thing happened every night when I was on call: I would be woken from my sleep to attend a mother with complications. The midwives would tell me, 'this lady has been in labour for 24 hours, she's now been pushing for two hours and the baby's stuck'. I would do a vaginal examination and find that the tissues were congested and swollen around the baby's head, the baby's head was squashed and moulding, and all around it was oedema (water retention creating an obstruction). It was ghastly and the only option was to apply forceps and drag the babies out. I think I was quite a skilled operator and tried to be as gentle as I could, but this situation necessitates an episiotomy and I despaired of having to carry out this procedure on women night after night.

Birth Story: Pasha

It was a Sunday morning when I awoke with the knowledge that Maya – my first daughter – was coming. It was a wonderful sensation of just knowing. I paced the house beaming 'my baby is coming'. I called Gowri and she came over at 11am. She examined me – I was 3cm dilated and purring like a fat, happy cat. Gowri talked me through a relaxation process, helping me to access the knowledge that I was safe and well, that my body knew exactly what to do; that I would just be opening, slowly and gently, ready to give birth at the hospital that afternoon.

My husband went ahead and prepared the birthing pool at the hospital, and we followed him when I was about 6cm dilated. On arrival, the midwife asked me how dilated I thought I was. I told her 6cm or so, but she laughed and said she would be very surprised – that I looked far too relaxed to be that far dilated.

To her surprise I was 9cm and my daughter was born within eight hours of the first contraction. She was a very relaxed baby, only crying when hungry. Her first months were spent arms spread out, palms up, completely relaxed, open and trusting in everything. I feel sure this is because of her peaceful birth.

I came to the conclusion that the underlying problem for a lot of these women was the mechanical fit. If you had a smaller baby, and a fit mother with an uncongested pelvis, it would be easier for the baby to pass through the birth passages. I was aware that in China, for example, women working in the paddy fields commonly squatted down and delivered their babies within the hour. Why? The reasons are simple enough. By squatting and rising as they work all day, they naturally encourage their baby into the optimal foetal position, and this exercise also aids lymphatic drainage within the pelvis and increases their pelvic mobility. But crucially, they also eat a wholefood diet of rice and vegetables, so their bodies are clear of toxins and supple. The importance of diet in the equation is highlighted by the fact that in developing countries that have adopted western diets and lifestyles, the number of caesareans and medically-assisted births has risen. Diet is the deciding factor.

However, it was 15 years ago that I came to this conclusion and voiced my concern that we were over-feeding mothers here. Not surprisingly, everyone thought I was crazy at the time and I met with a lot of hostility. There was a huge fear that babies would be born small. However, such scepticism proved unfounded – over the years my mothers have delivered babies of very healthy weights, usually 7lb plus. My emphasis was, and is, simply on having babies in keeping with the mother's frame. Today the 'eating for two' mindset is becoming redundant, as people are much more aware that a pregnant woman only needs an extra 200 calories per day – that's only an extra bowl of cereal per day.

I remember very clearly one mother who was admitted to the delivery suite in labour. She was a Filipino lady who was naturally petite – she can't have been any taller than 5ft – but she was grossly overweight. She had been in labour for 18 hours and was still only 3–4cm dilated. The baby's head was high up, her whole uterus was like a mound and the labour was clearly not progressing any further. I enquired about her diet and learnt that, since coming to England, she had started eating food that was alien to her native diet – such as bread, sausages and pâté – and she'd been eating too much of it. The result? She had to have a caesarean to deliver an 11lb baby when, according to her frame, she should have had a 6–7lb baby.

Invariably, whenever I was presented with mothers with huge abdomens and cervixes that wouldn't open and I asked about their diet, they would list their preference for comfort foods: 'Oh I had nausea and couldn't eat anything but toast', or 'I was addicted to chocolate'. This led me to think about dietary deficiencies, such as magnesium or chromium, which can lead to cravings. Soon I was beginning to think like a nutritionist.

What effects do certain foods have on our bodies? Wheat, for example, is known to create water retention. The first thing most nutritionists advise when present-ed with a patient complaining of neck tension and headaches, is to eliminate wheat from their diets. Eight times out of ten, the headaches disappear. Given that pelvic oedema is very often the underlying cause for inconsistent labours, I reasoned that wheat could be the culprit, congesting the vaginal tissues and restricting the cervix from gently opening and widening. I became even more convinced when I started asking about the birth experiences of women diag-nosed with coeliac disease. These women simply cannot eat wheat or gluten and although there has been no formal study into this, my own interviews with some of these women revealed that they enjoy incredibly short labours.

Sugar is problematic too. Sugar is metabolized via the Krebs cycle – the name given to the biochemical process that releases energy from the molecules of sugar. Studies have shown that a large number of free radicals are released during this process. The body finds it hard to neutralize these and they attack connective tissues like muscles, tendons and ligaments. When you are pregnant, you need your pelvic ligaments to be extremely supple and flexible, so avoiding sugar and sugary foods can prevent toxins being deposited in your uterus, cervix and pelvic structures.

Since my eureka moment 15 years ago, I have refined my nutritional guidelines into simple rules that are neither aggressive nor dangerous. Of course, there are times when that cake has your name on it, or it's difficult to resist the convenience of grabbing a sandwich for lunch. You're absolutely right, it can be difficult resisting the 'forbidden foods' on any diet, let alone whilst pregnant when cravings are enhanced. And of course there will be days when you feel frustrated, angry, or resentful at being forbidden from eating what you want – especially if, as is likely, you've grown up with the received wisdom that pregnancy affords you a guilt-free opportunity to eat whatever you like.

But when the sugar's calling, try to remember this. By buying this book you have already exercised your desire for a beautiful, blooming pregnancy and a gentle, controlled labour – and it is something you can achieve with focus, commitment and belief. Ultimately, no one else can do it for you and if you do cheat, you cheat only yourself.

So think positively. I like the old epithet: 'Rob Peter to pay Paul'. Compromise now for reward later. You've got just 35 weeks to follow this diet and get your body into tip-top condition and pristine 'birthfitness'. It's not so long in the grand scheme of things and you'll thank yourself afterwards. After the birth, my mothers always tell me how glad they are that they followed the eating plan.

Asian Culture and Pregnant Mothers

In South Indian and Sri-Lankan culture – which I was brought up in – it is customary for close relatives on both sides of the family to visit a pregnant mother regularly and take her some prepared food. Feeding a pregnant mother is considered to be one of the most meritorious acts in the Hindu religion and women within the extended family take pride in sending food to the pregnant mother. This time-honoured tradition gives practical support to the mother and enables her to rest, giving her a break from cooking. It also acknowledges the pregnancy and shows that the extended family has already begun to care for the unborn baby.

I tell all my mothers that you don't need to be Indian to follow this tradition. If your mother, mother-in-law, sister or best friend lives nearby, perhaps they could each cook you one meal a week. It can free up a valuable few hours for you in the evenings, particularly if you are still working. Just subtly give them your diet guidelines first – you don't want them turning up with a meal that has taken hours to prepare but is unsuitable for you.

General Dietary Guidelines

Below you will find lists of both foods to avoid and foods you should actively look to include in your diet. For brevity's sake and so as to keep the number of Dos and Don'ts being issued to you at a minimum, you will find that this list is not comprehensive. As a general rule, where a food has not been included on either list, you can assume it is okay to eat it, but be guided by your common sense as to whether or not it is suitable for this programme. Above all, the most important list to abide by is the Foods to Avoid section.

Foods to Avoid

Fruit: bananas (mucus-producing), grapes and mango (very high in sugar), citrus fruits

Wheat: bread, pasta and cereals made from wheat

Sugar: cane and refined sugar, fizzy drinks and fruit squashes, sugared cereals, chocolate, biscuits, cakes, puddings (if you have a sweet tooth you can have 2 teaspoons of honey per day)

Vegetables: restrict cooked tomatoes, reduce consumption of aubergines and potatoes, and eat raw salads, spinach and beetroot greens in moderation.

Both in Ayurveda and in the Microbiotic diet lightly steamed vegetables are regarded as highly superior to raw vegetables. This is because plant cellulose is digested in your gut by bacteria and this can release large quantities of gas. Once vegetables are cooked it is easier for the bacteria to digest them. In addition to this, in pregnancy the pancreas slows down its secretions of digestive enzymes. So to avoid abdominal distention and discomfort it is advisable to eat steamed or lightly cooked vegetables.

Meat: preserved meats, sausages, pâtés, pork and red meat

Fish: tuna has recently been given a bad press because of high levels of mercury found in its flesh (as a result to industrial waste dumping in the oceans). The metabolism of the tuna collects the mercury wastes easily and this can be passed on to the baby through the placenta, so it's best to avoid it while pregnant.

Foods to Enjoy

Fruit: pears – the royal fruit, lots of calcium; pineapples – for digestion; apples; peaches; nectarines; plums; avocado; apricots (high in iron)

Caution: have only three fruit portions a day. If you are eating dried fruits, try to choose unsulphured ones and count it as part of your fresh fruit quota. In addition to whole fruit, you may have ⅓ of a glass (150ml) of pressed or squeezed fruit juice a day.

Carbohydrates: rice (preferably brown), corn pasta, oats, barley, lentils

Vegetables: cooked greens, marrows, cucumber, carrots, parsnips and, as a general rule, any local vegetables that are in season (as long as they are not on the 'avoid' list)

Meat: chicken and occasionally lamb

Fish: with the exception of tuna, all types of fish are good. Oily fish like mackerel and salmon (preferably organic) are particularly important because they contain omega-3 oils (see box below).

Omega-3 fats

It is important to make omega-3 fatty acids a regular part of your diet for the following reasons:

- They help foetal brain and nerve tissue development.
- They help boost your metabolism, immune system and skeletal system.
- They are good for the brain, helping to elevate your mood and improve memory. They can even help stave off cravings for carbohydrates.

Omega-3 fatty acids can be found in oily fish such as anchovies, herring, mackerel, salmon, sardine and trout. Try to eat such fish three times a week at least. However, because of concerns about mercury and other contaminants in deep-sea fish, pregnant mothers may prefer to buy the fish oil supplement MorDHA, which has been filtered and chilled to remove mercury and other toxins. A vegetarian alternative is to get your omega-3 from oil: hempseed oil, walnut oil, flaxseed oil (also called linseed) or from seeds: pumpkin seeds, walnuts, flaxseeds. The oil or seeds can be sprinkled over foods such as cereal. (Note: Flaxseeds (linseeds) are very hard, therefore either grind them lightly (a coffee grinder is good for this) or soak them overnight.) You need about one large tablespoon of the oil or seeds a day. You can also buy the oil in capsule form. Recommended brands are: Mother Hemp Oil (hempseed oil), flaxseed oil, or Dr Udo's oils. (For stockists of all sources of Omega-3 supplements see Appendix C, page 312.)

Note: Flaxseed oil is the world's richest source of omega-3, containing double that of fish oils. The essential fatty acids omega-6 and omega-9 are also beneficial and are often found with omega-3 supplements. The ideal proportion of these oils is 3:(omega-3):2(omega-6):1(omega-9). This perfect combination is found in hempseed oil.

Nutritional and Herbal Supplements

As well as following the dietary guidelines outlined above I also recommend that mothers take nutritional supplements to maximize nutritional status and aid digestion. This is especially important during pregnancy as the digestive system is under a lot of strain during pregnancy and this can result in problems like constipation, heartburn, reflux and so on.

I recommend that every pregnant mother should take the following supplements:

- A general vitamin, mineral and trace element supplement. These are widely available and called 'Pre-natal' or 'Pregnancy' vitamins. Solgar and Biocare are the brands that I recommend.
- Probiotics are the helpful bacteria in the gut that break down the cell walls of vegetable matter and make the goodness within more accessible for digestion and absorption. They are available as capsules or tablets (Biocare and Dr Udo brands are good) and should be taken twice a day, half an hour before meals. Alternatively probiotic drinks and yoghurts from supermarkets can be taken if they are sugar-free and well within their sell-by date.
- Herbs are also an important part of this programme and I recommend my mothers have two different sets of herbs. These help prepare your body for a gentle birth and should be taken daily throughout pregnancy from week 13. These come in the following forms:
  - Herbal Tea
    Ingredients: false unicorn root, squaw vine leaves, cramp cut bark, raspberry leaf. This tea detoxifies and tones the uterus. Place one teaspoon of the above mixture in a teapot then add one pint of boiling water. Let it steep for 10 minutes, then strain and drink slowly. You can drink it all in one go or half in the morning and half later (just warm it up). It can look an alarmingly large volume to drink but many of my mothers come to really enjoy it.
  - Baladi Choornam drink
    Various Ayurvedic herbs are included in this powder (for stockist details see Appendix C, page 312). The powder is mixed with ½ a cup of warm

milk (goat's milk or rice milk is preferable to cow's milk as it's more digestible). It should be taken after your evening meal. This is started at week 13 of pregnancy. The herb Bala, the main ingredient of Baladi choornam, has the following properties:

– It reduces the undesirable effects of nervous excitability within the pregnant mother
– Has a calming effect on the central nervous system
– Regulates blood pressure
– Regulates the hormones of pregnancy
– Controls blood sugars thereby helping you to eat healthily (eating healthily can modulate your baby's weight)
– Very mild diuretic
– Stimulates regular bowel movements
– Softens the cervix and pelvic tissues

In addition to these herbal drinks, you should also take a tiny pill of herbs called the Dhanwantaram pill – I call them 'baby pills'. These contain potentized digestive herbs that are good for your digestion and absorption of nutrients and, as such, they help to nourish you and your baby. (See Appendix C, page 312 for stockist details.)

Dose: 1 a day along with your herbs.

Homoeopathic Tissue Salt Programme

During pregnancy the baby requires certain salts, which it gets at the expense of the mother. This programme will help to make good any salt deficiencies and help the baby with its salt requirement. Some health food stores sell tissue salts alongside their homoeopathic remedies, or alternatively try companies that supply homoeopathic remedies via the internet (see Appendix C, page 312). Alternatively, the Homoeopathic Tissue Salt Programme is available from the Jeyarani clinic.

Remedies:

Calc. Fluor. – for bone development and elasticity of connective tissue (helps prevent stretch marks)

Mag. Phos. – for heartburn and nerve development

Ferr. Phos. – for blood oxygenation

Nat. Mur. – helps control salt and therefore fluid balance, and helps prevent swollen ankles

Silica – for teeth, bones, hair and general strength

Dosage:

Take one tablet of each twice a day, morning and evening. The potency is 6c. If you are lucky enough to have a homoeopathic pharmacy nearby, they will combine the required tissue salts into one tablet for you – in which case take one twice a day.

Month 2 & 6	Month 3 & 7	Month 4 & 8	Month 5 & 9
Calc. Fluor.	Calc. Fluor.	Calc. Fluor.	Calc. Fluor.
Mag. Phos.	Mag. Phos.	Nat. Mur.	Ferr. Phos.
Ferr. Phos.	Nat. Mur.	Silica	Silica

Pregnant mothers may also like to take the following supplements:

- Digestive enzymes. I recommend Biocare or Dr Udo's digestive enzymes as a digestion support for mothers with abdominal distension and discomfort. Take one with breakfast and one with your main meal.
- Ambrotose. In the late 1990s a Nobel Prize was awarded for the discovery of 8 non-calorific sugars that make up cell membrane receptors for cell to cell communication. In nature all these 8 essential sugars should be available to us through the food that we eat; however, due to the storage of fresh produce and undesirable modern farming methods the food we eat is lacking in some of these nutrients. During pregnancy they are important for the development of the foetus and help the pancreas to normalize maternal insulin production and reduce the risk of gestational diabetes. Ambrotose can be obtained from Jeyarani (Appendix C, page 312).

Birth Story: Quick Labour Christine

On Sunday 12th September 1999, my contractions began at 5.00am. I visualized and meditated until they were 5 minutes apart, and decided to go to the hospital. My due date was the 20th September, so this was a week early.

We arrived at the hospital at 11.30am, where I was found to be 2cm dilated. We were told it could be early evening before the baby came, so we asked to be left alone so Mark could help me with breathing techniques and visualizations. He also massaged my back and big toes, especially during the longer contractions. Suddenly at 2pm, I had an almighty urge to push. Mark dashed off to find a midwife who was astonished to find that I was fully dilated. At 2.10pm, Logan Tyler Harris made his appearance, weighing 7lbs 15oz.

I'm proud to say that I took no drugs, had no tears, cuts or stitches and am recovering rapidly. I'm blessing my good fortune at having met Gowri, having heard many 'horror stories' about labour and the delivery.

Thanks to Gowri I could cope with labour and manage the whole procedure. I'm so grateful for the preparation that I learnt by attending her classes.

Ayurveda and The Gentle Birth Method

Ayurvedic remedies and philosophies feature strongly in The Gentle Birth Method. Ayurveda is an ancient system of medicine that has become fashionable in the West in recent years, but it is an automatic reference tool for me – something that I grew up with which complements my conventional medical training. Literally translated, Ayur means 'life' and Veda means 'science'. In India, where this 'life science' has been practised for thousands of years, it is a deeply respected and credible medical authority but I am particularly drawn to its holistic approach, especially its emphasis on emotional – as well as physical – caring for the pregnant mother and her unborn child.

Ayurveda groups the study of gynaecology, obstetrics and paediatrics together in a section of text called Kumara Bhritya, meaning 'how to take care of the child' and it draws a clear link between the mother's well-being and the health of the embryo, including its impact on the implantation process, early foetal development and the whole pregnancy.

Ayurveda expounds that the character, physical attributes and health of a child begins with the mother and her pre-conceptual status – in terms of how well nourished, rested and emotionally prepared she is for pregnancy and mother-hood. It also emphasizes the great need for the mother to be surrounded by the love and care of her partner. These values all align very closely to my own instincts about how we should care for expectant mothers and it is for these reasons that I allude to Ayurvedic wisdom throughout the programme.

Yoga is also an intrinsic part of Ayurveda and forms an important part of birth preparation. The section on exercise (see pages 75–83) outlines the benefits of yoga in pregnancy.

Ayurveda as a Diagnostic Tool
Ayurveda isn't just a support system for my own beliefs. It is also a great clinical guide and its teachings on constitution and body type are used in my programme in order to further eliminate pregnancy symptoms and rebalance the body for birth.

In fact, these guidelines are so detailed and accurate that whenever a new mother enrols at my clinic, I can tell within moments the problems she is likely to encounter during her pregnancy. There's nothing magical about it. In fact, many of you will be familiar with the physiological names given to physical builds – mesomorph, ectomorph and endomorph. Ayurveda works on a similar model.

In Ayurveda your body constitution is called your 'prakruti'. Each person's prakruti is composed of three body humours, or doshas, called vata, pitta and kapha. These represent a combination of the elements – water, air, fire, earth and so on – that, according to Ayurveda, make up the human body. Each dosha is responsible for different functions and parts of the body (see box below) so we each have all three doshas, although one or maybe two usually dominate. The dosha that dominates gives rise to a person's prakruti, which governs their physical and emotional characteristics.

If a person lives a healthy life according to their 'baseline' prakruti (at birth) then they can remain healthy and in balance – as long as they do other things to keep themselves healthy, such as exercise and avoid drugs and too much alcohol. However, many people do not live healthy lives and their normal levels of vata, pitta and kapha become unbalanced, which can lead to ill health. In pregnancy particularly, there are sets of symptoms that each prakruti will be susceptible to, hence, by identifying which body composition you are, you can further tailor your diet and lifestyle to prevent some of the related problems.

So What Do Vata, Pitta and Kapha Govern?

Vata represents wind and movement. It governs motion, activity and sensory functions; it controls the activities of the nervous system, blood circulation, contraction and expansion of the lungs and heart, intestinal peristalsis and elimination, and the contractile process in muscle.

Pitta represents fire and heating. It is responsible for all digestive and metabolic activities, regulating digestion and the secretions of the exocrine glands and the endocrine hormones.

Kapha represents liquid and cooling. It provides the static energy (strength) for holding body tissues together. It also provides lubricants at the various points of friction.

If any of the doshas become too dominant then the processes outlined above can cause complications.

On the following pages I have provided a basic breakdown of Ayurvedic principles, which you may find interesting and useful for more detailed diagnosis of how best to manage your pregnancy. However, whilst I am able to accurately use the Ayurvedic model in clinical practice, it takes many years to become an expert in the intricacies of Ayurveda, and it is not the aim of this book to list them here. I have kept the categories as simple as possible, but for those readers who still feel there is too much new information to absorb, stick to the general dietary guidelines at the beginning of this chapter. If, on the other hand, you are intrigued by the depth of an Ayurvedic assessment, I strongly recommend a personal consultation with an Ayurvedic practitioner, who can offer more comprehensive and accurate guidance.

Prakruti Analysis

Read each of the following statements and score them individually on a scale of one to five according to how accurate they are for you (0 = completely inappropriate, 5 = an accurate description). Add up the scores for each section – vata, pitta and kapha – and analyse the final scores to find your predominant dosha. Remember, the chart is a rough guide.

	0	1	2	3	4	5

Vata

I am slim and don't gain weight easily	
My appetite is irregular	
I have an erratic lifestyle	
I am a dreamer and don't usually finish projects	
I have irregular bowel movements and am prone to constipation	
I get cold hands and feet	
I am talkative	
I get anxious and worried easily	
I am creative and like to express myself creatively	
I prefer warm weather	
My skin is cool, rough and dry	
I am not very strong and lose stamina easily	
I walk quickly	
I am a light sleeper	
I learn easily but I also forget easily	
I get a lot of wind	
I am moody	
I find it difficult to make decisions	
I have short bursts of energy	
My menstrual cycles are irregular and I have period pains with associated headaches	
VATA TOTAL SCORE	

Pitta

My dreams are in colour	
I eliminate my food quickly through my gut	
I have a good memory	
I grasp things very well	
I prefer cooler climates	
I can be bossy and forceful	

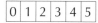

	0	1	2	3	4	5

I become irritable if I skip a meal	
I eat quite a lot	
I sleep soundly	
I have regular bowel movements	
I have good stamina for physical activities	
I am a perfectionist	
I don't like hot environments	
I sweat a lot	
People consider me very stubborn and I get angry very easily	
I criticize others and myself easily	
I have a very busy life	
I have a medium build	
My eyes are sharp and bright	
I like ice creams and cold drinks	
PITTA TOTAL SCORE	

Kapha

I am of big build	
I am muscular	
I prefer warm weather	
My hair is thick and lustrous	
My appetite is good and I enjoy food	
I learn slowly, but I have a good long-term memory	
I have slow digestion; this makes me feel heavy after a meal	
I walk with slow, measured steps	
I like a relaxed life	
I have regular bowel movements	
When I menstruate I have regular, normal periods	
I gain weight easily – people call me plump	
I have a pleasant voice	

	0	1	2	3	4	5

I am calm by nature	
I love sleeping and sleep deeply	
My skin is cool and oily	
I don't like cold weather	
I am good-natured and nothing seems to bother me	
I am possessive	
I wake up slowly and I don't like waking up	
KAPHA TOTAL SCORE	

Your highest score indicates your dosha predominance. You could be a vata, pitta or kapha mother. I have described each type of mother below and provided advice on working with your predominant dosha in order to restore balance and optimum health. You may find two scores are very close – as many people are a combination of doshas rather than one distinct category – but regardless of how close the score, follow the guidelines for your dominant dosha.

Vata Mothers

Typical Characteristics
- Lean, small frame
- Dry skin
- Mentally excitable
- Weak constitution – prone to colds and illnesses
- Poor circulation
- Poor digestion with tendency to constipation
- Low energy
- May experience fainting

Vata in balance: alert and spontaneous
Vata out of balance: worried and experiences mood swings

During pregnancy
- May show signs of clinical anaemia.
- May feel mentally slowed down, sometimes leading to depression.
- May experience aches and pains all the way through pregnancy.
- May experience nausea in early pregnancy.

Note: Vata is often heightened during pregnancy, regardless of which prakruti you are.

How to Counteract Vata
Exercise
- Exercise in moderation, as the vata mother is rather weak – engage in mild to moderate exercise only.
- Walking and swimming are good.
- Do indulge in some form of exercise – it has a mood-elevating effect.
- Avoid going to the gym, especially in the first three months of pregnancy.

Food
- Eat 3 to 4 regular light meals a day that preferably contain a representation of all the tastes like salty, sour, bitter, sweet, pungent and astringent.
- Avoid snacks in between meals.
- Choose clear soups.
- Avoid mushrooms.
- For non-vegetarians, chicken soups are recommended.
- Fish is also good if you can tolerate it.
- Avoid cheese as vata mothers have poor digestive power, especially in early pregnancy.
- Baladi choornam (my Ayurvedic formulation) is very good for vata mothers.

Herbs

The following herbs can balance vata:

- Black pepper
- Dill seeds
- Cumin seeds
- Basil leaves
- Parsley
- Ginger

Music

- Relaxing and calming music is very good for balancing vata.
- Chanting is beneficial. Many cultures and different religious persuasions use chants (see pages 82–3 for some mantras). The Gayatri Mantra is non-denominational.
- If you are religious, and depending on your religious leaning, you may like to recite prayers, such as the rosary, or Buddhist or Benedictine chants that instil peace and harmony.

Physical Treatments

- Massage with oils can be amazingly effective in reducing excessive vata.
- Self-massage or being massaged by your partner on a regular basis, for 20–40 minutes, is recommended. Suitable oils are virgin olive oil, or sesame oil.
- Essential oils can also be used to reduce vata – try lavender, rose, or jasmine oil. Use from 4 to 10 drops in 20ml of a base oil. This can be used for self-massage or by a practitioner during general or Creative Healing massage.
- Reflexology reduces vata, calms the mind and gives mental clarity. It also improves digestion and speeds up gut motility, thereby relieving constipation.

Vata Labour Issues

Factors to consider during delivery:

- The pelvis is usually smaller.
- The nervous disposition of vata mothers means they may experience more pain if not prepared effectively for birth.

- Lots of preparation, both mental and physical, is needed to avoid surgical intervention.
- Lots of low-back massage as preparation for labour will facilitate a manageable labour and gentle birth.
- Vaginal oils and stretching techniques as preparation for birth are invaluable in preventing instrumental delivery.
- Vata mothers need continuous massage during labour. Oil massages on the back, neck, shoulders and lower limbs are very beneficial during labour.
- Vata mothers are more prone to having a retained placenta. This is not a big problem and doctors routinely administer an injection that forces the body to expel the placenta. However, many of my mothers – aiming for a natural birth – are not keen to submit to drugs at this late point in their baby's birth, so in my self-hypnosis classes in London, I talk the mother through a hypnotic sequence in which she visualizes her body producing a surge of oxytocin (the hormone that encourages contractions) 15 minutes after the birth of the baby, thereby expelling the placenta. I have found this technique to be very effective on my vata mothers. If you are a vata mother, you can guide yourself through a short visualization of this hormonal occurrence – one or two minutes a day will be enough. You don't need any medical expertise to do this – simply by suggesting this automatic hormonal production whilst your mind is deeply relaxed and receptive, you can pre-condition your body to expel your placenta within 10–15 minutes after the birth.
- Vata mothers can have longer labours due to poor expulsive forces during labour i.e. poor uterine contractions, or uncoordinated uterine action, which can lead to slow dilation of the cervix.

Pitta Mothers

Typical characteristics
- Skin redness
- Medium-size body frame
- Slightly oily skin
- Fluid retention

- Angry
- Mentally irritable and edgy
- Quick tempered
- Intolerant of others' behaviour
- Experiences skin burning sensations
- Feels too hot all the time
- Can't tolerate hot weather
- Hates closed environments
- Prone to feeling faint
- Prone to increased sweating
- Good memory
- Sound sleeper

Pitta in balance: perceptive and intense
Pitta out of balance: angry, impatient and frustrated

During Pregnancy
- Prone to bleeding in early pregnancy
- Prone to post-partum mental problems
- Excessive appetite
- Can have semi-solid stools

How to Counteract Pitta
The remedy is to cool and calm everything down.

Exercise and Lifestyle Changes
- All gentle forms of exercise, e.g. gentle swimming or gentle tai chi, would be beneficial. Pitta mothers must take care not to increase their heart-rate by more than 110 beats per minute as this can aggravate pitta.
- Walks with your partner. Walking in the moonlight is specifically recommended in the Ayurvedic text because it cools you down.
- Pitta mothers need a lot more love and affection than other mothers.

Food

- Avoid hot and spicy foods like pepper, chillies, garlic, vinegar, salad creams, pickles and sour things in general.
- Acidic foods are heat-producing as a general rule and this aggravates pitta.
- No alcohol as it causes your system to heat up, aggravating pitta.
- Avoid foods that are too hot in temperature.
- Avoid cheese as it is very difficult to digest.
- Most vegetables are good – cucumber, marrows and pumpkins are ideal; beetroots and carrots are very cooling and recommended.
- Eat melons as a separate meal – they need special enzymes from your pancreas to digest them. Eating them with other food puts a huge strain on your digestive system.
- Eat grains such as rice, millet, corn and oats in moderation (not more than 1 small cup of any of these cooked grains per meal).
- Try to cut out tomatoes. If you must eat them restrict it to only once a week. Tomato is very acidic and can cause aches and pains. Cooked tomato is worse than raw tomato.
- Coconut is very good for reducing pitta. The white kernel and coconut milk, which is extracted from the white kernel, can be used for cooking. However, use only small amounts of coconut in your cooking, as it is high in fat.
- Apples are very good.
- Avoid citrus fruits as acidic food increases pitta.
- Having a banana once a week can reduce pitta. As a general rule I do not recommend them as they are too fattening and mucus retentive.
- Vegetable soups with herbs are very soothing.
- Congee, an overcooked broth of rice with water and salt, is very easy to digest. To make it more interesting, a little garlic or ginger and a few vegetables can be added to it.
- Milk is cooling and is good for reducing pitta. Ideally it should be goat's milk – try to avoid cow's milk unless it is labelled with the A-2 protein as opposed to A-1. The A-1 proteins that are found in the herds of some cows produce undesirable effects in the human digestive system and have been associated with gut problems (specifically colon cancer), coronary disease, diabetes

mellitus (Type I), multiple sclerosis and autism. In the near future, it will be possible to segregate the cows that produce A-2 milk from those that produce A-1 milk. This will be done by a simple test on a hair of each cow. (A-2 milk is already on the shelf in Australia and New Zealand.) Closer to home, Guernsey cows produce A-2 milk. However, Jersey cows produce A-1 milk, so if you are buying milk look for pure Guernsey cow milk. (This was reported on BBC Health News, 9 April 2001.)

Herbs
- Choose cooling herbs like coriander in food.
- The herb Bala (*Cida codifolia*), a main ingredient in my Baladi Choornam drink, is very important for keeping pitta under control.
- Shatavari (*Asparagus racemosus*) is another popular Ayurvedic remedy that can reduce excessive pitta, however, it must be taken under the supervision of an Ayurvedic physician.

Treatments
- Creative Healing massage includes a cooling procedure that is good for counteracting excessive pitta (see Normalizing Body Temperature, page 57)
- For massage, use essential oils like lavender, jasmine and sandalwood. The recommended base oils for pitta are sesame oil and coconut oil.
- Have a milk bath as Cleopatra did. Simply add some milk into your bath water (cow's or goat's milk).
- Take a flower bath, with petals of flowers floating in the bath. Try rose or jasmine flower baths.
- Use meditation to calm the mind.
- Listen to gentle and calm music.

Pitta Labour Issues
Factors to consider during delivery:
- Labour tends to be shorter than average.
- High blood pressure can develop during labour. This must be monitored – if pitta is highly out of control it may lead to eclampsia.

- If there is increased pitta, it can lead to bleeding during delivery of the placenta.

It should also be noted that pitta mothers are more prone to post-natal depression. This can be prevented by keeping to the pitta protocol for diet and treatments.

Kapha Mothers

Typical characteristics
- Large frame
- Oily skin
- Gains weight easily
- A tendency for water retention
- Drawn to sweet foods
- Digestive sluggishness
- Passive
- Calm, steady
- Lethargic
- Slow to be irritated
- Heavy sleeper

Kapha in balance: strong and calm
Kapha out of balance: dull and lethargic

During pregnancy
- Can experience aches and pains in the joints and spine.
- May experience breathlessness.
- Prone to gestational diabetes – even the baby can develop diabetic tendencies.
- Indigestion is common.

How to Counteract Kapha
Exercise
- All forms of exercise benefit the kapha mother. Aerobic activity such as walking and swimming are ideal for boosting oxygen supply to the body and

to the baby, and for supporting the heart, which is under more pressure during pregnancy. But keep an eye on your pulse and make sure your heart is working at no more than 120 beats per minute. Yoga and stretching build strength in the muscles, encouraging them to protect the mother's skeletal structure. But avoid all twisting exercises and do not use your abdominal muscles at all, as they will have separated to allow room for the baby. Pilates classes should be avoided for this reason, but are excellent for post-natal recovery.

Food

- Do not eat anything white or pasty – so avoid toast, bread, rice pudding and all puddings.
- Avoid pasta, cakes, sweets, crisps and ice creams.
- Avoid beef, pork and lamb. Chicken is allowed – two small portions per week.
- Choose spicy foods.
- Eat lots of green vegetables and light clear soups.
- Fruits to enjoy: apples, apricots, cranberries, pears.
- Vegetables good for kapha include: asparagus, celery, leafy greens, spinach, turnips, coriander, parsley.
- Kapha-predominant mothers can also eat chicken, eggs, fish, goat's milk.
- Eat pumpkin seeds, sunflower seeds, flax seeds.
- Don't over-cook grains; eat when just done.

Treatments

- Warm baths are very beneficial. To make the bath more therapeutic you can add a few drops of essential oil of basil as this activates your endorphins and improves your mood.
- Other essential oils that can reduce kapha and lift your mood are eucalyptus, camphor, neroli, tea-tree, juniper and fennel. Use in massage oils, or add a few drops to your bath.
- In Sri Lanka and India, it is common to add medicinal leaves called Nirgundi to your bath. The botanical name of Nirgundi is Vitex Nirgundi. In ancient

Ayurvedic texts this is prescribed to reduce kapha. It is best to use fresh crushed leaves. Alternatively a tincture can be obtained (see Appendix C, page 312).

- Have regular lymphatic drainage massages (Creative Healing massage is very efficient for lymphatic drainage).
- Alternatively, a simple self-massage can be given with dry finely powdered mung beans. The powder acts as a fine abrasive and as an astringent to draw out excess body fluids. A pinch of medicinal turmeric can be added to the mung bean powder. Triphala powder can also be used in powder massage; this is a powder made up of three fruits that suit all doshas. (Mung bean powder can be made yourself by crushing them in a coffee grinder to a fine consistency. Medicinal turmeric and Triphala powder can be obtained from any Ayurvedic supplier – see Appendix C, page 312).
- Warm oil massage can be incorporated with powder massages. Triphala oil is available and this can be mixed with sesame oil and used for massage. This can be done as a simple self-massage all over the body with circular strokes, or it can be performed by an Ayurvedic technician. The Triphala oil and sesame oil can be obtained from any Ayurvedic supplier.
- Reflexology is very good for reducing kapha. Focus on the lymphatic drainage reflex areas on the feet to make sure that the lymph drainage channels are kept clear. I recommend at least ten reflexology treatments from 20 weeks of pregnancy to term.

Kapha Labour Issues

- Kapha mothers usually experience uncomplicated deliveries.
- If kapha is not controlled during pregnancy the pregnant mother gets the classic 'bloated' look. Excess kapha means that the progress of labour can be sluggish with longer labours. Moreover, the baby can get stuck (due to congestion and oedema in the cervix and the pelvic tissues) and the mother may need a Caesarean.
- Kapha mothers are prone to going past their due dates, if their excess kapha is not remedied in pregnancy.

Gentle Birth Method Recipes

Over the years, I have had many mothers come to me worried about what to eat and what not to eat. I fully appreciate that it can be daunting to work from both my own dietary guidelines and the Ayurvedic recommendations for each dosha, so I have slowly accumulated a roster of appropriate tasty recipes. A selection of these recipes, which are suitable for all doshas, can be found in Appendix A (see page 277).

Birth Story: The second-time mother – Annabel

I was thrilled to discover I was pregnant with my second child, but once the elation subsided, I felt a deep sense of dread and fear. Would the birth be as traumatic as last time? Would I have to go through induction, stitches, infection and post-natal depression again? As the months went by, I became increasingly anxious. A friend gave me an article about Dr Motha and despite being very sceptical about anything that might be considered 'alternative', I decided to go and see her.

I had very little idea of what to expect and was startled by Gowri's positivity. One of the first things she did was take a full history and actually listen to me explaining my first birth experience. It was a huge relief just to have someone calmly listen, let me talk and not try to explain away or belittle what I had felt. After that, Gowri's approach was to assure me with absolute confidence that my experience need not be repeated.

I saw Gowri about five times before the birth and felt much more physically and mentally prepared than I had previously. One of my biggest concerns was that I would again need to be induced and suffer bad tearing.

I was two weeks late and there didn't seem to be much sign of an arrival, so my husband and I decided to go for a long walk. We trudged for hours up and down hills and even though nothing happened, just being outside in the fresh air seemed to help my mood.

When I got home I had a hot bath and as I got out, my waters broke. I was really excited and pleased – already I had managed naturally part of the birth experience, which I had begun to think was not going to be possible for me.

A few hours later I was still in a state of high excitement but there were no contractions. We went to the hospital and saw the midwife, who said I could go for another 24 hours before they would want to induce. She recommended another walk. The time, it was in the freezing February rain, and was unpleasant. We got home and I began to think induction was inevitable, when at about 4pm, my contractions started. I felt a huge rush of excitement and fear.

After about an hour, I put on the TENS machine and the contractions started coming closer and closer together, with increasing power. I spent a lot of my time on all fours, crawling about or leaning against the walls. I phoned the hospital at about 6pm and was told to delay coming in for another couple of hours, or until I was unable to walk.

Suddenly, the contractions began to feel very painful indeed and I had the first sense of an urge to push. We got in the car and drove to the hospital. By the time we got there, I was crawling on all fours. The midwives examined me and I was 7cm dilated. I asked to get into the birthing pool and felt an immediate sense of relief at being in the warm water. It felt comforting and made my body seem supported. I used gas and air as well, and this also helped me to relax. At this point, the pain was terrible and I felt overwhelmed. I was desperate to push even though it had only been a few minutes since my last examination. However, when the midwives checked me again, I had gone to full dilatation.

Within a few minutes, the baby's head had crowned and the contractions had become more regular and less frightening. The midwives told me when to push and within the next few pushes the head emerged, followed quickly by the rest of my daughter's body. I got out of the pool and was immediately handed the baby, and the placenta was delivered. I was checked and, to my amazement, told I had no need for any stitches. All my greatest hopes for the birth had been fulfilled. I had a beautiful baby girl that I had pushed out without assistance in the water, and I had not torn.

The midwives then ran me a bath and the next hour was spent gazing at our daughter, breastfeeding and absorbing the experience we had just been through. Over the following weeks, I found that in contrast to my first birth I was left feeling elated and empowered. I was amazed at the speed of my recovery, there were no stitches, no complications and the bruising cleared within a few days. I found I was able to cope much more easily with everything.

I know that Gowri's help made an enormous difference to my second experience of birth. I was mentally and physically prepared and although the birth of my first child made me apprehensive, Gowri's approach enormously reduced the fear I felt and gave me the confidence to enjoy a natural birth. I now feel very strongly about the benefits for all women of following Gowri's advice and, in particular, her mental and physical preparation techniques. I am currently awaiting the birth of my third child and I have once again found Gowri's support invaluable in preparation. I just wish that all women were routinely offered the kind of care and support that she has given me.

The Gentle Birth Method Treatments

One of the most important factors in the success of The Gentle Birth Method is that it helps eradicate many of the problems encountered during pregnancy – such as back pain, nausea, heartburn, fluid retention and so on. Much of this is due to the intensive therapies included in the programme. As well as being heartily welcomed by my mothers for the 'pamper factor', these therapies are a quick and effective way of rebalancing the body and tailoring it into optimum condition for the birthing process. In a nutshell, The Gentle Birth Method makes the mother birthfit in all 3 realms: physical, mental and emotional.

The Origins of the Treatment Programme

As the number of women presenting congested vaginas and enormous babies continued to rise, I realized my role as a Senior Registrar meant I was simply becoming an expert in crisis management. By the time I became involved in the mother's care, there was rarely anything I could do to help them, except intervene with forceps, ventouse or scalpel. It saddened me and was not why I had entered the profession. Every birth is a miracle, and should be a personal triumph for every woman. Why was it so rapidly becoming something fewer and fewer women could achieve without help? I fully believed doctors and the medical establishment should be investigating preventative measures that would help women prime their bodies for birth, before they went into labour. The diet I devised was certainly a step towards helping women control the size of their babies and condition their bodies for birth – but it wasn't a coping mechanism for the realities of labour. It came as a flash to me that all I needed to do was to create a total birthfitness programme and to make the mother birthfit so that they could have the gentle birth they wanted. Hence I began researching front line treatments that would boost the detoxifying effects of the diet but also help with pain management.

It was at this time that Michel Odent conducted the first waterbirth, in Pithiviers general hospital near Paris in France. The idea of mothers delivering their babies in water excited my interest. When an opportunity to meet Odent came up, I jumped at the chance and learnt what clinical conditions he created for the waterbirths.

It all sounded quite simple, but knowing the hospital wouldn't indulge my 'fancies', I purchased a pool from my own pocket and put it in a room at the far end of the obstetric corridor in Whipps Cross Hospital. I instructed the midwives – some of whom clearly thought I'd lost my marbles – to let me know of any mothers who were interested in the idea of a waterbirth and soon a few did come forward. Imagine my frustration then, when after a few hours of staying in the pool, they would politely ask to go back to their rooms.

It was clear that sitting in the water in itself wasn't enough to reduce the pain of labour, nor to shorten it. So, with a group of seven mothers – I call them my 'pioneer mothers' – we started some self-hypnosis classes, incorporating visualizations and learning how to breathe and relax, thereby adding a mental element to the birth preparations.

At the same time, I was approached by two reflexologists, Mary Martin and Helen Chittick, who volunteered their services to the antenatal clinic on a Friday afternoon. The benefits of reflexology in helping certain medical conditions, such as high blood pressure, were already well documented, so I was willing to refer mothers with high blood pressure to be treated with reflexology. In every single one of these cases, the mother's blood pressure went down. Word quickly spread through the clinic and I started getting mothers presenting with different problems. I remember one mother in particular, who had developed severe Diastasis Symphysis Pubis in her pregnancy (DSP causes severe pubic pain and instability as the pubic joint begins to separate under pressure from the pregnancy and the influence of pregnancy hormones). Her condition was so painful that she couldn't walk and had to use a wheelchair. However, after just three reflexology treatments, she was able to get out of her wheelchair and walk again. I was very impressed.

Along with this clinical antenatal success, we made another startling discovery – those mothers who had received reflexology treatments delivered their babies in much shorter times. Some mothers were delivering in 5–6 hours, as opposed to the commonly observed 18-hour labours. One 46-year-old woman delivered within a few hours of being in labour, which made me realize that it's not your chronological age that determines your birth experience, but your biological age. A toxic lifestyle – i.e. smoking, alcohol, junk food and a lack of exercise – can make the tissues of a woman in her twenties function rather poorly; conversely an older mum can function amazingly well physiologically if she commits to a healthy lifestyle with optimum nutrition and a physical fitness programme.

The Power of Touch

Have you noticed how nearly everyone you meet is compelled to touch your bump? People almost can't help themselves. A baby bump is intrinsically soothing to the human psyche and even those who wouldn't presume to kiss you in greeting, reach out their hands to share – for a fleeting moment – the joy of contact with an unborn child.

The power of touch is well documented. Our bodies surge with feel-good endorphins when we are stroked and caressed, boosting our immune systems, dulling our responses to pain and even contributing to a longer life. And the good news is this effect is enhanced yet further during pregnancy. Your increased blood volume not only contributes to a blooming complexion, strong nails and glossy hair, but also means the tiny blood vessels beneath your skin are positively tingling for touch.

Throughout this book, I will show you and your partner how to use touch in a myriad of ways – for example, to deepen self-hypnosis, bond with your baby and reduce your chances of a vaginal tear. A lot of the recommended treatments are technical procedures and require a qualified therapist but, where possible, I've adapted certain massage techniques so that you can do them at home. In some instances, you can do them on yourself, although it is best if your partner becomes involved in the treatments. I would like to think that most of you reading this book will share the advice on these pages and work together as a unit – as a family.

Even before birth, you can nurture your baby into a relaxed and loved little individual. Whenever your partner massages you, he is soothing his baby too. Remember, your baby receives physiological support from you on a continuous basis and also picks up on all your feelings. So, when you feel loved and supported by your partner, so does your baby, absorbing all your endorphins. In turn, special hormones that are released from the baby's placenta prepare you for the birth process and motherhood. A ten-minute massage by your partner not only relaxes you but sends a wave of fresh, nourishing oxygen to the womb and placenta. It's an intimate opportunity for you to snuggle up as a family and pass on thoughts of love and safety to your baby – what more powerful incentive can there be to make every day of your pregnancy as happy, stress-free and precious as possible?

So surrender to the treatments I list on these pages – they're not cosmetic treatments, all have a direct physiological effect on your birthfitness: realigning your joints, super-boosting the detoxifying effects of the diet and moulding your muscles to become loose, pliable, soft and flexible for birth. Just as importantly – you'll feel pampered in the process!

The Father's Role

Did you know that as a father you are also expecting? If you thought the bump/cramps/pain bit was the mother's domain, think again. OK, so you're not going to grow a bump, you're not going to be woken with leg cramps in the middle of the night and, no, you don't need to go through labour – but pregnancy is not something that just happens to the mother for nine months. Having a baby is a shared adventure.

You don't suddenly become a father when the baby finally emerges. You're a father already. From the moment you see the little shape on the ultrasound monitor and see the smile on your partner's face, you can start bonding with your baby. The comic view of the expectant father is of a desperate man driving around at 2am trying to find pickled onions to satisfy the mother's cravings and desperately trying to put up shelves in the nursery as the male nesting instinct translates into frantic DIY. But your role in pregnancy doesn't just have to be practical stuff and 'doing' things.

Your body may not be engaged in pregnancy, but your heart and mind can be. Your baby, growing inside your partner's belly, already recognizes and loves your voice and your touch. And for your partner too, your role in the pregnancy is absolutely crucial. Feeling looked after and cared for is a powerful tool in the mother's emotional preparation for birth – the more she learns to trust and rely on you for support, the more she will instinctively feel safe surrendering her body and freeing her mind from the mechanics of labour.

So when your partner asks you to read to her a visualization that involves imagining the inside of her pelvis, or to help her build up an emotional dreamscape for her 'safe place', be enthusiastic. Knowledge is understanding, is empathy, is sharing, is bonding – is family.

You may know every last curve of your partner's body but by reading this book you can also learn about how she is growing your baby. Become an expert, a connoisseur of her body. Read its messages, anticipate its demands; love, nurture, cherish it – and in so doing, you love, nurture and cherish your baby. Whatever your relationship history up until this point, pregnancy is a new chapter that offers opportunities to be a better partner and the best father.

Father's Tip: Belly bonding

It has been proven that a baby in the womb can distinguish its father's touch from an unfamiliar hand on the mother's tummy. So take every opportunity to stroke your partner's belly, talk to your baby and play touch games (like 'round and round the garden...'). You may feel silly doing this while your baby is still in the womb but your baby knows it's you and it's an invaluable opportunity to start bonding.

Touch Tips

- Exchange gentle oil massages with your partner. These are instant body boosts that will calm and relax you. Add 2–3 drops of lavender oil to 20ml of base oil (for example, olive or sunflower oil) and take turns massaging each other's feet for 10 minutes each evening. This helps relax the whole body and is a caring way to bond as you prepare for parenthood.
- Share oil baths together and softly stroke your 'baby bump'. This soothes and relaxes the baby, as well as nourishing your skin, keeping the skin elastic and supple, and preventing stretch marks.

Your Baby Keeps You Young

Your baby will help keep you young. In India, my grandmother always told me the age you are when you become a mother, is the age you stay. Of course, she meant emotionally, but there is some physical truth in it as well. Cosmetic companies have long been aware of the replenishing properties of placental hormones and growth factors, and use them in anti-ageing programmes and skin rejuvenation creams. Science has shown that the baby's placenta produces growth factors that circulate into the mother's bloodstream. Hence rejuvenation is a natural gift from the baby to the mother!

Overview of the Treatments

Reflexology
What is it?

Reflexology is a unique system of therapeutic foot massage that targets precise reflex points. It is based on the premise that the feet are mini maps of the body and every reflex area on the foot relates to a vital organ in the body. The philosophy behind the treatment is that life force, or prana, circulates in a balanced, rhythmic way throughout the body. If this energy is disrupted, say by an injury, then signals are transmitted down energy channels, within the body, to the feet. Here they manifest as thickenings, or tiny nodules that feel like grains of sand, in the reflex areas of the feet that correspond to the area of injury on the body.

Its pedigree

Reflexology has an esteemed history. Like acupuncture, it has been used in China and India for over 5000 years. In Egypt, ancient hieroglyphic drawings have been found that depict royal persons receiving reflexology with the caption 'you shall thank me for the pain' (when the nodules are massaged to break down the granules it can be painful). There is also evidence that Native American tribes knew of the relationship between the reflex points and the internal organs of the body and used this knowledge to treat disease. Reflexology has been steadily assimilated as a complement to conventional Western medicine since the 1870s, in the fields of dentistry, gynaecology, chiropractice, chest medicine, orthopaedics and ENT. In addition, it is now being used in a growing number of other specialities within UK hospitals and in general practice clinics within the NHS.

Reflexology in pregnancy

My inclusion of reflexology in the initial pregnancy strategies that I developed was accidental, yet it is now one of the most powerful tools in my programme. You may find, as you have more and more treatments, it helps to identify areas within your body that need cleansing. Many of my mothers find their feet are indicators of their internal health and enjoy finding out how the reflex areas are improving with reflexology as the weeks go by. As mothers progress through their pregnancies, they are quick to point out specific areas of tenderness in their feet that correspond to a physical weakness elsewhere, such as a tender sciatic nerve.

Reflexology is very safe in pregnancy, and is instrumental in helping 45.5 per cent of my mothers give birth at the optimum gestation of 40 weeks. At term, it can be effective in initiating contractions and labour by stimulating the pituitary, adrenal and uterine reflex areas.

Note: In the early weeks of pregnancy (up to 12 weeks), before the placenta is fully established, I generally advise a gentle foot massage, concentrating on light drainage and working only on the upper areas of the foot. Along with this I recommend positive visualization and Reiki. In the month-by-month guide on pages 131–83, there are specific indications for reflexology at different stages of pregnancy.

What it can do for you in pregnancy

- Reduce and normalize high blood pressure (hypertension). Weekly treatments of reflexology for 30–45 minutes usually reduces high blood pressure and can help you avoid repeated admission to hospital for rest and observation
- Normalize low blood pressure
- Eliminate oedema and reduce swelling in feet and ankles
- Prevent heartburn
- Improve sleep quality
- Clear headaches
- Relieve varicose veins
- Clear pelvic congestion
- Improve lymphatic drainage and complement the effects of the recommended eating plan

- Aid digestion by boosting the pancreatic secretion of digestive hormones – the pancreas can become sluggish during pregnancy due to the effect of the placental hormones
- Oxygenate the baby by improving the blood flow within your whole body, your uterus and the baby's placenta
- Help you to carry your baby to term
- Can be used to initiate labour if you are overdue, thereby reducing the need for medical induction at hospital
- Intensify contractions during labour and shorten labour as a result

Can you do it yourself?
Yes, partly. Below is a basic five-minute massage that can be performed on the feet or hands.

Method: A light all-round kneading of each foot can help to relax your whole body. Specific lymphatic drainage is encouraged by working deeply on the tissues on the top of the recipient's foot by moving your fingers up and down the spaces between the bones and massaging deeply. (The same techniques can by applied to your hands – simply massage up and down the webbed area between the fingers on the top of the hands.)

Birth story: Reflexology benefits during labour – Tricia

My contractions started at 12.15am and were every 20–30 minutes. By 6am they were every 5–10 minutes and by 9am, every 3 minutes. I arrived at hospital at 9.45am and was found to be 6cm dilated. By 1.00pm, I was fully dilated. My waters broke at 1.15pm and Robert was born at 2.36pm.

Throughout the contractions, I concentrated on my breathing and other than occasionally walking around, I knelt on the bed, holding

---

41

the headboard, rocking backwards and forwards in time with inhaling and exhaling.

During the birthing process, I sat upright so that I could push downwards. Other than four gasps of entonox, I had no pain relief, other than my husband massaging my feet. I did notice that when he massaged my feet, the contractions weren't so severe.

Creative Healing
What is it?
No this is nothing to do with mystic powers, it's a specialized hands-on massage technique using virgin olive oil. Its aim is to restore function to a disturbed part of the body. This is achieved by applying the four principles of Creative Healing, which are:

1. to normalize body temperature through cooling or warming techniques
2. to create drainage channels to decongest (along with lymphatic drainage)
3. to remove congestion by light massage on thickened areas under the skin
4. to reposition displaced substances i.e. within vertebral disc spaces, or knee cartilage.

Its pedigree
Creative Healing was developed by Joseph B. Stephenson, who was born in 1874 in Newcastle upon Tyne, England. He migrated to America, where he practiced as a respected healer for over 20 years and passed on his method to several chiropractors and physical therapists on his retirement. Creative Healing has a wide following in the United States and in 1989 I met Patricia Bradley of The Joseph B. Stephenson Foundation of Creative Healing, based in California. Struck by the simplicity and effectiveness of the method, in 1990 I invited Patricia and her husband John to come to London to teach us the method. Since then I have been practising Creative Healing and have taught courses in England, Europe and India.

Creative Healing in pregnancy

The success of Creative Healing in clearing the body of congestion and optimizing physiological function was my primary reason for incorporating it into my Gentle Birth Method programme. There is a great need for the joints and muscles of the lower back, sacrum and coccyx to be functionally mobile and clear from congestion if a mother is going to have a gentle birth. When muscles and ligaments within the body are returned to their natural state, they automatically become supple and elastic. The Creative Healing treatments in the programme concentrate on bringing about this transformation to the birthing areas – the spine, pelvic area, sciatic area and sacrum. However, since birth is a function of the whole body, treatments for the organs that are important to maintain optimum health – for instance, the heart, liver, pancreas and gut – are included at specific times during pregnancy.

What it can do for you in pregnancy
- Reduce nausea and vomiting
- Optimize digestion and pancreatic function
- Relieve constipation and regulate bowel function
- Increase energy levels
- Reduce breathlessness
- Reduce anxiety and stress
- Eliminate back and neck pain
- Eliminate sciatica
- Stimulate the lymphatic drainage in all key areas of the body
- Cleanse and drain the pelvic area

Can you do it yourself?

Some parts. The basic General treatment explained on page 55 can be administered to you by your partner. This is gentle and easy and has immediate benefits. However, the most important massage technique for your partner to learn is the Pelvic Drainage massage (see page 68). This is a 10-minute procedure that ideally should be performed every other day, especially from 36 weeks of pregnancy, in order to create more space for your baby's descent into your pelvic birthing space.

You will need to see a qualified Creative healer for the other treatments that tone up your heart, digestive system and other vital areas of your body.

Creative Healing glossary

Although it's unlikely that you had ever heard of Creative Healing before embarking upon The Gentle Birth Method, my guess is that Creative Healing will quickly become one of your favourite elements of the programme. But even though it is profoundly relaxing, this comprehensive massage treatment can leave mothers boggled at the range of different treatments on offer. Many mothers ask me why they have to have a heart treatment or a pancreatic treatment for instance, when a general back treatment would feel just great. Hence I've compiled a glossary that explains why you receive such specific treatments and what they achieve at different stages of your pregnancy. As I told you at the beginning of this book, there's a physiological intention at the root of every physical treatment you receive on the Gentle Birth Method – and that can be easy to forget when it feels so good.

General treatment: (also known as the General Lymphatic Treatment)
This is an essential initial treatment that is done prior to any other Creative Healing treatment and sets up drainage in the whole of the body to clear toxins quickly.

Heart treatment: In early pregnancy, the heart treatment is given to help the heart cope with the dramatic increase of 30 per cent in circulatory blood volume of the mother. The heart treatment is also received just before delivery, because the cardiac muscle is called upon to work hard during labour. Occasionally, pregnant mothers complain of palpitations and feelings of unrest surrounding the heart and the treatment can help to reduce this. These symptoms are often attributed to mental anxiety and fear. A heart treatment is also advised post-natally.

Hiatus hernia treatment: Offered alongside the heart treatment, it helps with reflex oesophagitis (heartburn) and is also effective in calming the feeling of nausea during pregnancy.

Pancreatic treatment: This treatment has been found to be excellent in improving digestive function. As well as insulin and other hormones, the pancreas secretes important enzymes to help with the digestion of food. The symptoms in pregnancy associated with the digestive system – such as nausea, heartburn, abdominal bloating and constipation – have been reported to improve after a pancreatic treatment. In the programme, it is recommended at 32 weeks to prevent gestational diabetes from developing, as the placental hormones might suppress insulin response at this time.

Lungs: Creative Healing is effective in treating chest infections in pregnancy by clearing the drainage channels. This is not a standard treatment and is only given if a patient is suffering from a chest infection.

Liver: This is very helpful in early pregnancy when many mothers suffer from nausea and vomiting. Often, these symptoms are related to high levels of circulating tissue toxins that clog up the liver and slow down its detoxification mechanism. A liver treatment can clear these symptoms. This treatment is usually carried out at set times throughout pregnancy.

Thyroid: The thyroid is challenged during pregnancy and mothers tend to feel more tired if the thyroid function is compromised.

Kidneys: The kidneys are responsible for clearing excess tissue fluids and it is important to keep them functioning well.

Spleen: This treatment offers immune modulation and helps the white and red blood cells to be formed and released at an optimum pace.

Back and spine treatment: Spinal health is of paramount importance as all the nerves that transmit impulses to the muscles of the limbs and trunk originate from the spine and emerge through spaces between the vertebrae.

Abdominal toning: Digestion and assimilation of food is vitally important in maintaining the health of mother and baby. General abdominal toning realigns the energy flow to all of the abdominal organs. It is offered throughout pregnancy and before treating any of the organs within the abdomen. Mild abdominal pain and diarrhoea caused by a tummy bug can be eased with abdominal toning.

Pelvic drainage: This upwards and outwards massage is applied on the lowest part of the abdomen just above the pubic bone. It directs excess fluid away from the pelvic floor area and also decongests the cervix and tissues within the birth canal.

Sacrum drainage and sacro-iliac treatment: Started early in pregnancy, this ensures the sacrum is able to move and mould as the baby's head drops down into pelvis as pregnancy advances. These treatments clear congestion and loosen the sacro-iliac joints. This helps the mother greatly during the second stage of labour, shortening the pushing time. Constipation is also effectively treated with a specific 7-minute treatment on the sacral area. There is also a 10-minute sacrum treatment that treats haemorrhoids.

Sciatic treatment: This treatment is for alleviating the classic symptoms of sciatica, i.e. pain radiating from the mid-buttock down the back of the thigh and the leg, all the way down to the toes. There is a special nerve centre on the sacrum that can be centred in order to prevent sciatica occurring at any stage of pregnancy.

Bowen Technique
What is it?

During a Bowen session, specific areas of the body are subjected to gentle rolling movements that subtly disturb and reposition the muscles. Bowen initiates a physical change because the muscular disturbance (from the rolling movements) is emitted through the central nervous system to the brain. In response, the brain sends a command to the muscle to reposition, helping to eliminate any previous inflammation or stiffness in those soft tissues.

Its pedigree

This technique is named after Tom Bowen (1916–82), the Australian therapist who developed it. As a young man in the 1950s, he regularly visited the clinic of a local man with an excellent reputation as a 'manipulator', watching him work and listening to what he had to say. Bowen developed his own technique on the back of this apprenticeship, and opened a clinic treating a wide range of injuries, illnesses and disabilities. In the 1970s, the Australian Government Report into Complementary Therapies found that Tom Bowen had successfully treated 13,000 people.

Bowen in pregnancy

I find that the gentle nature of the Bowen treatment helps to instil emotional calm, an attribute that is particularly important during pregnancy. My mothers tend to love the profound relaxation that it gives. It is also non-invasive. I find it invaluable for treating acute conditions like pubic pain and other musculoskeletal pain.

What it can do for you in pregnancy

- Relieves back pain
- Relieves sciatica
- Relaxes the pelvic ligaments and muscles and helps pelvic mobility – this helps the baby's head to engage in the pelvis
- A gentle manoeuvre on the coccyx can help initiate labour if you are over-due

Can you do it yourself?

No. This technique must be carried out by a qualified therapist.

Reiki

What is it?

Reiki is a therapy in which energy is transmitted, via the laying on of hands, to key areas of the head, face, trunk and limbs. The treatment can be given through normal clothes, so it is non-invasive.

Reiki warms and relaxes the body and facilitates gentle healing by attracting lymphocytes (the immune system cells) to the affected area. It is a very still treatment and for those who like something more dynamic, it can feel as though nothing is being done – but healing is happening, just on a subtle level. It is very common to feel deeply relaxed and even fall asleep during the session.

Its pedigree

In the early 1900s, Dr Mikao Usui, a Japanese Christian theologian, was allegedly given the secrets of healing in a vision he had following a 21-day meditation and fast. His teachings were passed down and have spread through-out the world. Once initiated, a Reiki practitioner may get immediate results, however it takes many years and hours of dedicated practice to channel the Reiki energy in a more powerful way. The early Reiki masters were able to heal advanced diseases effectively.

Reiki in pregnancy

Reiki can be received at any time during pregnancy, as it is so gentle and safe. It is one of the safest treatments you can have in early pregnancy.

What it can do for you in pregnancy

- Improve quality of sleep
- Deepen muscle relaxation
- Instil calm and reduce anxiety before the birth
- The stillness and peace that is part of a Reiki session can give you mental space to accept pregnancy and bond with your baby

Can you do it yourself?

Yes – to a limited extent. Simply laying your hands on someone with healing intent will have a positive physiological effect. It has been proven that if you place your hands on any part of the body, the electromagnetic energy and warmth of your palm attracts lymphocytes (the intelligent part of your immune system) to the area and this can encourage healing. However, positive intention is all-important.

Cranio-sacral Therapy
What is it?

This is a 'light-touch' technique that fine-tunes the body's rhythms. The therapy is based on a subtle pulse, the Cranio-sacral rhythm, which moves through the core of the body – through the brain and spinal cord and the fluids that bathe them. The pulse has a tide-like rhythm that becomes irregular where there's a blockage or restriction.

These blockages – often characterized by tightness – are usually the result of the body holding so-called 'tissue memories' of a stressful event, such as a physical injury or a traumatic emotional situation. By freeing the restrictions in the connective tissue and muscles through Cranio-sacral therapy, we can bring about the release of tight ligaments and muscles, realign joints and even release emotional stress.

Following a session, patients will very often feel increased warmth, tingling or energy surges.

Its pedigree

The cranio-sacral pulse was discovered by a team of neuro-surgeons and neuro-physiologists. They observed subtle movements of the dura (membranes covering the brain) during brain surgery and came to the conclusion that restrictions of this pulse could cause functional disorders. Cranial therapy was then evolved to restore optimum movements of the cranial bones and the cerebro-spinal pulses.

When the egg and the sperm fuse at fertilization the subtle rhythm of life begins and the pulsations of the embryo are immediately visible. This is later seen in the cranio-sacral rhythm, in the membranes that surround the brain and in the circulation of the cerebral spinal fluid.

Cranio-sacral therapy in pregnancy

Cranio-sacral therapists believe our life histories – including our emotional and physical traumas – are 'held' in our bodies. Hence the release of tension in the joints and muscles also releases tissue memory and emotional stress. This therapy can therefore calm and soothe all mothers.

The therapy also helps prepare you for the birth process. The therapist checks the movement of the sphenoid bone at the base of the skull, which houses the pituitary gland. This gland lies just below the hypothalamus and both the pituitary gland and the hypothalamus are responsible for producing and releasing prolactin and oxytocin, the hormones for pregnancy and birth. Through cranio-sacral therapy, the sphenoid bone is able to move freely, ensuring normal release of these hormones for birth.

What it can do for you in pregnancy

- As a preparation for birth it can release muscle and tissue restrictions that can prevent the pelvis from opening easily during birthing

- The circulation of cerebro-spinal fluid pulse is regulated and this helps with optimum releases of oxytocin during labour
- Can be used during labour to enhance contractions
- Alleviates emotional stress

Can you do it yourself?
No. The method of listening to the body's rhythms that is intrinsic to this procedure is very subtle and too specialized to précis. Visit a qualified therapist.

Vaginal and Perineal Stretch Massage
What is it?
A specially-devised massage that stretches and softens the lower vaginal tissues, preparing them for the delivery of the baby's head.

Its pedigree
Early forms of this technique have been routinely practised in India and Africa for hundreds of years. In India, the Ayurvedic preparation for birth includes a vaginal 'picchu', which involves inserting a medicated oil-soaked bundle of soft cotton into the vagina to soften the tissues. In Africa, a similar method is practised using herbs, combined with a vaginal stretching technique. They make a bundle of herbs and insert it into the vagina. The bundle size is increased as term approaches. (The herbs are sometimes wrapped in muslin). I have combined both methods and since introducing it to the programme, the incidence of vaginal tears in my mothers has dropped to less than 4 per cent.

Perineal stretching in pregnancy
This procedure is to be practised daily *after* 36 weeks – DO NOT DO IT BEFORE THEN. It is a very important part of the programme because it reaches the parts deep muscle relaxation cannot sometimes reach. Even if our limbs are limp, the vaginal muscles can remain tense – generations of tucking in our tails, pulling in our tummies, riding, dancing and walking have meant our vaginal muscles have evolved to be tight.

What it can do for you

- Create more space in the vagina for the delivery of the baby's head
- Reduce the second stage of labour (i.e. the pushing stage)
- Reduce the incidence of vaginal and perineal tears
- Reduce pain in the vagina and perineum during birth as the baby's head is born
- Reduce the sting or burning sensation of the crowning stage
- Maximize the elasticity of the lower vaginal muscles and tissues
- Soften the tissues around your vagina thereby reducing pressure effects of your baby's head and reducing bruising
- The distress experienced at the transition stage is often minimal or absent in mothers who practise the perineal stretch massage
- Observing your body's rapid response to the practice of vaginal stretching can increase your confidence in your ability to give birth
- Less bruising means quicker recovery after birth

Can you do it yourself?

I recommend that your partner performs this massage technique for you, but you can also do it yourself. The method is described in detail on page 69.

Case History: Perineal Stretch Massage

I remember a pregnant client of mine who in the past had done lots of Ashtanga yoga, and whilst the rest of her muscles and tissues felt soft and were incredibly relaxed, her vaginal muscles and tissues felt like rock. At the first perineal examination at 36 weeks her lower vaginal muscles would not budge at all when pressed. I sent her home with some oil and instructions on how to do the vaginal and perineal stretch massage but thought it would be too late to soften such hard tissues. Within just three days of using the oil and performing the self-stretch she herself reported that she had noticed a big change in her vaginal elasticity and by the time she gave birth, three weeks later, her

---

perineum was sufficiently soft to prevent any tearing at all – a great result despite a difficult start.

Home Massage Treatments

This section of the book is one of the most important. It really allows you to take charge and prepare your body for labour, rather than having to wait for your allotted time with a therapist. By performing these techniques at home, you can do them as often as you like (although no more than daily). I find many of my mothers really look forward to their treatments – and best of all, they're free.

Remember to reciprocate and perform some massages on your partner (although obviously not the perineal stretch!) as it is vitally important your partner feels cherished too. It's very easy for everything to centre on the mother, but these treatments can really help the father feel involved in the pregnancy.

Points for partners to remember (for the back, neck and tummy massage)
- If in doubt, apply a light touch to begin with and gently increase pressure, with the mother's guidance.
- When you begin a massage, muscles can tense up initially, so encourage relaxation by softly stroking and massaging the area. Don't go straight in with strong pressure.
- These Creative Healing massages are very light. The pregnant mother should avoid deep body massage, as it can release toxins and cause unpleasant symptoms such as headaches and nausea.
- Repetition is key. Massage is not about lots of different and dramatic moves. Even if you think it must be terribly boring for the mother, continue anyway. Drainage is maximized by repetition.
- Make sure your hands are warm.

Creative Healing Massage

As I pointed out previously, there are four 'intentions' in Creative Healing – to normalize body temperature, to open and create drainage channels, to remove congestion, and to reposition substance. However, each of these intentions is not necessarily appropriate to all massage treatments – for example, in a heart treatment there is no repositioning of substance, only drainage and the removal of congestion.

The techniques that are used in Creative Healing are explained below, followed by instructions on how to massage particular areas. (Note: A demonstration of the entire Creative Healing massage techniques on DVD is available from Jeyarani – see Appendix C, page 314.)

- Normalizing body temperature (cupping and taking the heat off)
  This does not relate to the body's own innate temperature, but to heat in the local site of congestion. To normalize temperature, first compare skin temperature by lightly touching the back of your hand across the area you're treating (the back of the hand is more sensitive to temperature differences). If there are any 'hot spots', cool them by cupping the hand and repetitively fanning downwards, without actually touching the skin – the aim is to create a 'cooling breeze'. However, if an area is much cooler than other areas, it should be warmed up by briskly rubbing down the skin with the palms of alternate hands using a drop of oil.

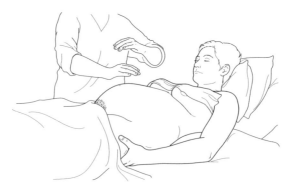

Example of Cupping and Taking the Heat Off

- Opening and creating drainage channels
  In Creative Healing drainage channels are created by making a superficial vacuum over the skin of the area to be treated. For example, downwards along the sides of the neck, upwards in the lower abdomen, across the chest for the heart, etc.

- Breaking down congestion
  To stimulate lymphatic flow in the area to be treated it is necessary to break down congestion. Areas of congestion feel like lumps or knots under the skin and these are broken down using little circular movements of the fingertips and thumbs.

- To reposition substance
  Disorders of body function can occur because nerve centres or cartilages are displaced in the body due to sudden movements. In Creative Healing, repositioning substance is part of the treatment in key areas such as the vertebrae, around the knee and shoulder joints and in the pubic area.

The General Treatment (Massage for the Neck, Shoulders and Back)
(General lymphatic treatment and muscle release for the whole back)
Minimum treatment time: 20 minutes

Benefits
- Deeply relaxing
- Reduces muscular tension in the whole of the back
- Facilitates lymphatic drainage
- Has amazing detoxifying effects
- Provides anxiety relief
- Increases musculo-skeletal mobility to shorten labour
- Encourages the baby's head to engage

The purpose of this light massage technique is to help stimulate the lymphatic system, to drain the tissues, reduce oedema (swelling) and help the muscles work more efficiently. It can be an ideal time for the mother to practise simple relaxation and visualization phrases (we will look at this in detail in the next section) so that she links feelings of relaxation with pleasant touch and hypnotic triggers. The birth partner can help her with this, saying softly and slowly: 'Take three deep breaths and whisper I'm going into self-hypnosis now', or 'Relax for me', or 'Let your mind drift to your safe place and feel safe there...' For this treatment all you need is *virgin olive oil*. Some mothers ask if essential oils can be added to this and yes, of course, you can add a couple of drops of good quality organic lavender essential oils to about 50ml of olive oil. However, it isn't advisable to complicate matters by adding a combination of oils to this, as the merits of Creative Healing are based on working on the energy lines and have nothing to do with the healing properties of essential oils (unlike Aromatherapy, for example).

The treatment is done with the *mother sitting upright* on a firm surface, such as a chair (sideways on, so that the back of the chair does not get in the way), stool, or bench. Note: All back treatments are done sitting up as lying down will close the spaces between the vertebrae and it will not be possible to treat the spine effectively. The mother's upper back is exposed, but she can hold a towel in front of her body to prevent feeling exposed or cold. It is important for you to feel comfortable as well, so find a chair to sit on while administering the massage. Start by standing behind the mother, make sure your hands are warm, then place them on her shoulders and be still for a moment.

During this massage the whole of the back is worked on, so for ease of understanding the back and spinal area is divided into three sections. (By the way, don't be put off by the medical jargon, it simply provides an accurate description of the spaces to be massaged.)

I) The upper back

This covers the neck area from the occiput (the base of the skull) down over the shoulder blade area to the area where a bra line would be.

Normalizing temperature

Using the back of your hand, sweep across the back and neck to identify 'hot spots' (or areas of congestion). When you find them, cup your hand and use the 'cooling breeze' to reduce the temperature in those areas (as described on page 54).

Opening drainage channels (alternate with *Removing Congestion* (see below))

To drain the lymph down the sides of the neck, use your three middle fingers. Place the three central fingers together with the middle finger slightly behind the other two, to create a 'trough'. The three fingers are then used to make downward sweeping movements from behind the ear, close to the bony prominence (the mastoid bone) down towards the base of the neck. On every third or fourth stroke, make longer sweeps that continue across the top of the shoulder. Start on either side of the neck and after about 12 or so sweeps, do the other side. Use your right hand to treat the right side of the mother's neck and the left hand to do the left side.

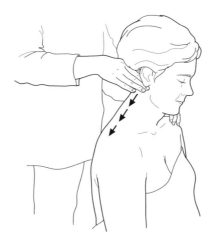

The General Treatment: Opening Lymphatic Drainage and Energy Channels

Identify the triangular clavicle space or hollow (called the supraclavicular fossa) created by the lines of the collarbone and the outer margin of the trapezius (or neck muscles). Within this area are lots of important structures such as blood vessels, nerve plexuses and lymphatics. The main lymph drainage channel is called the thoracic duct. This collects lymph all the way up from the feet to the chest. It traverses the triangular space above the clavicle and drains into the subclavian veins within the neck area. This massage will ensure good drainage so that toxins from the whole body are carried away.

Removing congestion and clearing the primary lymphatic filter area in front of the neck
Using the tips of the index, middle and ring fingers, make small, light circular rotations across this space, covering the edges too. Imagine your fingertips are searching for grains of sand in the tissue just beneath the skin surface. This can be done for a minute at a time, *alternating with the drainage movement down the sides of the neck* (above) – one side at a time. It is very important to use a light touch for this technique – it should be gentler than when working on muscle.

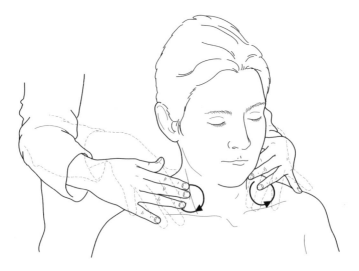

The General Treatment: Removing Congestion

For further drainage of toxins, cup your hands with the thumbs closed next to the fingers and create a slightly cupped shape with the palms of your hands. Place them on either side of the spine on the lowest part of the ribs. Now move your cupped hands up the back using small circular movements. You want the movement of your hands to be like a caterpillar (I actually call this movement the 'cupped caterpillar'), so you will find that as you move your hand the middle part of it will move closer and then further away from the back. During this treatment your intention is to create a vacuum and drain all the toxins over the shoulders into the triangular supraclavicular space in front of the neck.

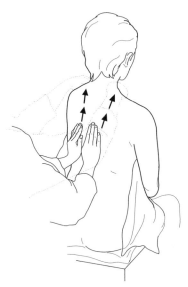

The General Treatment: the Upper Back (the Cupped Caterpillar)

To complete, once again clear the triangular space above the clavicle using little circular movements with your fingers as you have done previously.

If the shoulders feel tense you can alternate the cupped caterpillar movement with a feathering movement (small short circular strokes with the thumb, moving up the back) to help loosen tense muscles. The thumbs work across the muscles between the shoulder blades and spine, just gently teasing out the muscles (this can be done during the birth too, to help keep the mother relaxed and loose).

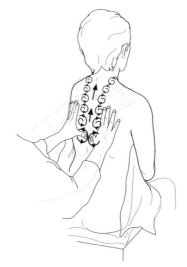

The General Treatment: the Upper Back (Removing Congestion)

Loosening the neck muscles downwards

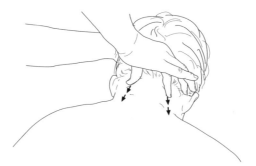

The General Treatment: the Upper Back (Removing Congestion and Draining)

The final part of treating the upper back and shoulders includes the loosening up and downward drainage of the muscles directly at the back of the neck at the midline, from the occiput (base of the skull), down to the last cervical vertebrae. Often these muscles feel like two solid columns due to muscle tension and the most efficient way of loosening these neck muscles is to work downwards in little circular movements using gentle but firm pressure of the thumb and forefinger of your right hand. These movements should be followed by draining straight down the vertical columns of muscle, with longitudinal strokes, using the same fingers. Alternate between the circular and straight-down movements. Finish by draining the toxins that you have released from the neck by using the cupped caterpillar movement from between the shoulder blades, up over the shoulders into the triangular (supraclavicular) spaces in front of the neck (as done earlier).

II) The middle back
This covers the area below the lowest part of the shoulder blades (around where the bra line would be) to the iliac crest (the rise of the hips).

Encouraging drainage
Cup the hands and make gentle, *downward flowing* strokes across the kidney area. As the hands approach the iliac crest, let them glide over the hips and travel under the bump, towards the pubic joint (below the front of the belly). This movement helps to encourage kidney drainage and pushes excess tissue fluid toward the lymphatic channels in the groin. Perform these movements for about 3–5 minutes.

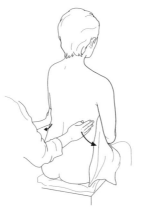

The General Treatment: the Middle Back (Lumbar Drainage)

III) The sacrum

Here you will be working on the sacrum and loosening up the sacro-iliac joints and the ligaments in that area. The sacrum is the upside-down triangle below the last vertebra.

Breaking down congestion

Locate the two 'dimples' of the sacrum with the thumbs. (If the dimples are not visible, place your hands on the top of the mother's hips and where the thumbs rest will be the approximate position of these dimples.) Make small upward and outward rotating movements with the thumbs in this area. It may feel quite nodular or lumpy so do check if the pressure is comfortable. Often the sensation is quite pleasant for the recipient, although the area may be tender. These movements help to make the sacrum more flexible, meaning it will open more effectively during the birth. It also helps the emptying reflex of the colon.

This massage can also be performed during labour, for 7 minutes at a time, and has been found to help both the mother progress to second stage more quickly, and reduce the length of the second stage.

Removing congestion on the sacrum and the sacro-iliac joints

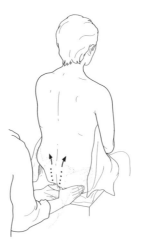

The General Treatment: the Sacrum (Removing Congestion on the Sacrum and Sacro-iliac Joints

Place your thumbs, with the thumbs pointing horizontally at each other, at the bottom of the sacrum really low on the coccyx (tailbone) in between the buttocks. Spread your hands flat over the lowest part of the buttocks. Hook the thumbs under the tailbone, if possible, and roll up a fold of skin and underlying tissue towards the top of the sacrum and the last mobile joint of the spine. First do this movement directly upwards and then gradually fan your thumbs outwards until you are working along the V-shaped sacro-iliac ligaments. Perform this upward stroking movement for about 5 minutes, with the intention of removing congestion. (Please note: the sacrum should be massaged only in an upward direction.)

This movement helps to decongest and loosen the sacrum, helping the baby's head to descend easily into the birthing space. It also increases the flexibility of the coccyx. Note: If this massage is performed regularly during the last few weeks of pregnancy, the baby's head is encouraged to engage deeply in the pelvis at 36–38 weeks.

Every so often you should repeat the 'dimples thumb massage' for a minute or two.

Occasionally, using cupped hands, drain horizontally outwards across the buttocks from the sacro-iliac ligaments, around the hips and to the front of the pelvic area underneath the bump. These movements help to loosen up all the muscles within the buttocks and increases pelvic mobility. Do this horizontal massage for 2 minutes at a time.

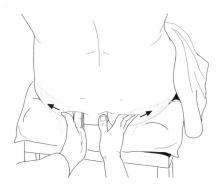

The General Treatment: the Sacrum (Horizontal Sacral Drainage)

Repeat the entire sequence of the above set of movements slowly over and over again until you get a sense of loosening (approximately 5 minutes).

As you become more practised at the method you may notice how the texture under the skin changes. If the skin seems puffy, it usually means that you need to work more often on breaking down congestion and drainage.

Please do the General Treatment massage of the neck and shoulders, upper back, middle back and sacrum as often as possible every week for about a total of 20 minutes. This assists the mother's back and pelvis to easily stretch and allow the baby's head to engage and be born through the inner diameters of the pelvis.

Back and Spine Treatment (Treatment for loosening back muscles, toning the back and back pain)

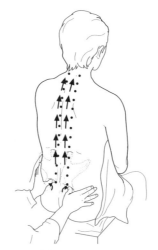

Back and Spine Treatment (Remoulding and Repositioning Substance between Vertebrae)

The Creative Healing back treatment is useful for treating back pain due to different causes. Even if there are no specific back problems this treatment strengthens the back and keeps it flexible, which is important for giving birth. The partner uses the tip of the thumb of each hand on either side of the spine to replace displaced substances in between the vertebral spaces. Most back pain is caused by the displacement of tissues: however, even if there is no displacement the back trouble can be helped by this remoulding movement.

The mother sits upright on a firm bench. Begin at the bottom of the spine, identify the lowest space between the sacrum and the last lumbar vertebrae – to find this ask the mother to rock gently forward and you will be able to identify the space between the sacrum and the last mobile vertebra of the spine. Place the tip of your right thumb horizontally in the soft space about an inch away from the mid-line on the right side of the spine. Feel your thumb gently sinking into this spot and with a light pressure rotate the thumb from a horizontal to a vertical position. Do not go beyond the vertical. Repeat the same movement in the same space on the other side of the spine using the left thumb. During the quarter twist of the thumb make sure that the thumb stays in the same spot. Once you have done this in the first space, move up the spine one space at a time, left hand following the right hand, until you reach the base of the neck. Work slowly with a healing intention. Once at the top of the spine use the palms of the hands stroking directly downwards, one following the other, straight down the middle 10 times. Repeat this remoulding using the thumbs as many times as you feel is necessary.

A valuable movement for remoulding the spine and loosening up tense columns of muscles on either side of the spine. The mother should sit up-right on a firm seat. [N.B. All back treatments are done sitting up as lying down will close the spaces between the vertebrae and it will not be possible to treat the spine effectively.] During this movement the thumbs are forming two blades of a pair of scissors, the rest of the fingers are stretched out and held together as units. The partner should start by placing the right thumb on the left side of the spine, with the tip of the thumb in the space between the sacrum and the last vertebra (fifth). The left thumb is placed above it on the right side of the spine in one space above the other thumb, so that the thumbs are crossing. The tips of each thumb form a pivot point. To perform the movement move the thumbs from the horizontal to vertical positions: if you think of your thumbs as two blades of pair of scissors, the scissors close. The thumbs in this way make a quarter turn in each space. Proceed in the same way up the entire spine to the base of the neck. Then begin again at the lowest part of the spine, this time with the left thumb in the higher position. These two upward movements are considered a 'set': perform 5-6 sets of these movements and then stroke downwards over the spine one palm following the other 10 times.

[Note: this movement loosens the back muscles and the vertebrae. I often describe this movement to my students as a bird flying up the spine.]

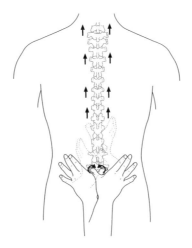

Back and Spine Treatment (The Scissors Movement)

Abdominal Toning

Abdominal Toning intends to realign the energy lines within the whole of the abdominal cavity and create a sense of harmony and balance between the digestive organs and the pregnant uterus with the baby within. In my experience this has a very beneficial effect on placental circulation. On our programme we routinely apply abdominal toning to all mothers from the time that they book onto our programme. (Note: On occasion a mother has been referred to me for intra-uterine growth retardation with reduced amount of amniotic fluid, and performing abdominal toning for 10 minutes followed by specific nutritional advice has often restored the foetal growth rate and amniotic fluid levels to normal.)

Benefits
- Oxygenates the baby
- Encourages lymphatic drainage of the contents of the whole abdomen
- Tones the uterine muscle and encourages placental circulation
- Decongests the veins
- Reduces swelling in the legs
- Helps with digestive function and grants the mother a sense of 'lightness' within the abdomen

Technique

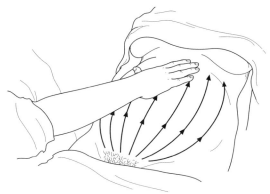

Abdominal Toning

The mother lies on her back on a bed, or couch, propped up on pillows at a comfortable 45-degree angle. Olive oil is used as a lubricant. The outer borders of the abdominal area are identified by the rib cage on the top and the bikini line on the bottom.

Sit or stand comfortably on the right-hand side of the mother. Start with a cupped right hand with an open palm with the thumb out at right angles to the rest of the fingers. Place this hand on the left hand side of the abdomen at the bikini line and sweep upwards in a straight line towards the ribs. Follow the curve of the bump. Once the thumb crosses the margin of the rib cage allow the thumb to close against the other fingers.

Then break contact and start again at the bikini line having moved a bit towards the midline of the body. Continue with these movements in close parallel lines until the right hand side of the abdomen is reached.

Repeat this sequence from right to left and so on for 10 minutes. Cool the skin as you go along (taking the heat off with your cupped hands).

Pelvic Drainage

This helps to remove excess fluid accumulation in the inner pelvic area, especially around the base of the cervix and the uterus. This kind of water-logging often buoys up the baby's head in the lower abdomen, delaying the baby's head from engaging and resulting in a longer first stage of labour.

Benefits
- Oxygenates the baby
- Decongests the pelvic area and tones the uterus
- Encourages the baby's head to engage
- Hastens labour
- Decongests the veins
- Reduces swelling in the legs
- Helps to calm cystitis

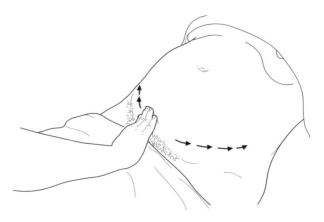

Pelvic Drainage

Technique

The mother lies on her back on a bed or couch, propped up on pillows at a comfortable 45-degree angle. Olive oil is used as a lubricant and the masseur (ideally the mother's partner) should warm the oil between his hands before applying it to the mother's abdomen. Again, he should start with a cupped right hand, drawing the palm of the hand from the midline of the pubic bone to the right, along the bikini line, underneath and up around the tummy towards the iliac crest (hip bone). This should be done with a very light touch (no pressure moves) 10 to 15 times. Now switch hands and switch sides to the left and do the same. In total it should take about 10 minutes. The masseur should cool the skin by cupping as he goes along.

Vaginal and Perineal Stretch Massage

This massage technique is one of the best things you can do to help yourself during your pregnancy. Be aware that you may feel some tenderness in the tissues as they are stretched for the first time, particularly if you are very athletic, a dancer or ride horses. All mothers find that the vaginal muscles are thicker and more rigid on one side than the other. This is often related to your walking pattern, with either a left- or right-sided dominant gait causing hypertrophy of one side of the pelvic floor muscles.

For this massage I recommend you use my special Ayurvedic Perineal and Vaginal oil, which has been formulated to soften the vaginal muscles (although olive oil can be used simply as lubrication). If you are using the vaginal oil, use this to soak 7.5cm (3in) of a 15cm (6in) long strip of sterile gauze about a centimetre thick and insert 7.5cm (3in) of it into your vagina. This should be in situ for four hours before you do the massage – this will help to soften the tissues. Remember to dispose of the gauze before doing your vaginal stretching!

I prefer partners to perform this technique on the mother, because someone else can get a better depth of stretch, particularly after 36 weeks of pregnancy when your bump may be so big that you might not be able to reach the lowest part of your vagina. However, you can do it yourself, so this is also explained below.

Benefits

- Creates more space in the vagina for the delivery of the baby's head
- Reduces the second stage of labour
- Reduces the incidence of vaginal and perineal tears
- Reduces the sting or burning sensation of the crowning stage
- Maximizes the elasticity of the lower vaginal muscles and tissues
- The transition stage is often minimal or absent in mothers who practise the perineal stretch massage
- Helps reduce the pressure effects of the baby's head, such as bruising, meaning a quicker recovery for you

Technique

Before you begin, make sure your hands/your partner's hands are washed clean and that the fingernails are short. Lie down with your back propped up at a 45-degree angle. Remove the gauze swab.

Your partner should insert one finger, up to the first knuckle, into the vagina.

Breathe in deeply and, as you exhale, your partner should gently press his finger back towards the coccyx. He should relax the pressure during your in-breaths and push back with his finger only when you exhale. This trains your tissues to relax open when you exhale, as you would push the baby out during exhalation. Repeat six times, then change direction.

The stretch is only done in three directions: directly behind, to the left side and to the right side – never to the front. Imagine the directions as being at 6 o'clock, 4 'clock and 8 o'clock positions within the lower half of your vagina. By the end of the first week, you will find a sense of 'give' in the muscles and you may progress to being stretched with two fingers up to the first knuckle. Eventually you will be able to insert two fingers deeper, up to the second knuckle, stretching more of the vaginal tissues.

If you are stretching the vagina yourself, you may find it easier to stand and prop one leg up at a time on a chair then reach down between your legs *from behind* and stretch your vagina with your index finger and middle finger. Change hands as you change your leg positions. Again, stretch the vagina at the 4, 6 and 8 o'clock positions towards your tailbone, within your posterior vaginal wall. Remember to breathe out as you stretch and relax your fingers as you inhale. Stretch six times in each direction and for maximum benefit, do this exercise every day.

Some of my enthusiastic mothers and fathers have impressed me with their dedication to stretching and have delivered 9lb babies without a graze!

I have to emphasize that even with preparation some mothers give birth more easily than others. It is my intention to motivate all mothers to prepare their vagina to the best of their ability, as this preparation is a great source of comfort. If you know that your vagina has been prepared to open generously and can cope with the delivery of your baby's head, without harming your tissues, you can then mentally relax when you are in the pushing stage of birthing.

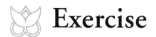 Exercise

Many pregnant women curtail their level of physical activity quite dramatically when they are pregnant – even those who were previously regular gym-goers. In the early weeks, this is understandable. After all, you're probably battling with exhaustion and most probably a litany of other complaints. Plus, the risk of miscarriage is considerably higher at this stage. Even though there is no evidence to prove that continuing with your regular exercise after you fall pregnant can lead to a miscarriage, it's understandable that many mothers feel more protective of their bodies – and more aware of the stresses and strains they place on it.

However, once you enter the second trimester, it really is paramount that you introduce – or continue with – a certain level of exercise. I'm constantly amazed at how little people consider the fitness that's required for pregnancy and birth. I don't recommend my mothers put on more than 20lbs during their pregnancy, but even that modest figure is a huge amount of extra weight for your body to be carrying around. This places great stress on your bones and joints, especially when you consider that your growing baby takes calcium from your system. This is why a reduction in bone density is common.

Many mothers say they feel 'like a beached whale', or a 'galleon in full sail' by the end of their pregnancy, unable to see their toes or tie up their shoes. But you don't have to feel enormous in those last months. After all, your bottom will never look trimmer as your rapidly expanding tummy dwarfs all your other contours!

The benefits of the wholefood diet mean my mothers don't put on large amounts of weight, but have a taut, round tummy – they're invariably considered to have a 'neat' bump. But I must emphasize that muscle tone is important too. It's such a shame to ruin a good pregnant silhouette with untoned arms for example – and you'll be thankful for stronger biceps when you're holding your newborn baby day and night.

As well as boosting your self-image, exercise and fitness makes your pregnancy more enjoyable because you will be more mobile – rather than being left stranded on the sofa, waiting for the big day. In fact, the exercises I advocate actually optimize your chances of a good birth, by 'cradling' the baby forward into the best position. This is known as optimum foetal positioning and encourages the baby to drop head-down into the pelvic cavity, with its spine running down the front of the mother's tummy. Known as the occipito-anterior position, it drastically reduces the incidence of back pain during the first stage of labour, and encourages effacement (thinning) of the cervix due to the pressure of the baby's head pressing down on the cervix.

Most importantly of all, you'll be thankful for your fitness when you go through labour. My first-time mothers average 10 hour 32 minute labours, and my second-time plus mothers average 5 hours 37 minutes. These numbers are lower than the national averages, but even if you can sleep through the first few hours, you've still got a long stretch ahead of you in which you'll be dealing with your contractions and battling the psychological pressure of anticipating how many centimetres you've dilated. It can be crushing to hear you've only dilated 2cm when you've been in labour for six hours and, if you work from the '1cm per hour' rule, you can find yourself looking at another eight hours of the same. Many women demand an epidural at this point – too exhausted to keep going through it all. Of course, you can remain upright and mobile to help gravity speed up and intensify the contractions but this takes enormous stamina when you're managing contractions. And if your labour starts during the night – as more than 60 per cent do – then you could be tired before you've even started.

I don't want these scenarios to scare you but rather to make the case for birth-fitness. Exercise isn't an optional part of the programme; it is a must. Labour is like a marathon. You could have six or more hours of intense physical activity – of managing contractions and pushing when you are fully dilated. It's not something you just turn up and do on the day – you have to train for it. Your body has to be conditioned, ready and at its peak. This programme makes you think about muscles you've never considered before – your uterus, your pelvic floor, we even think about your mind as a muscle – but let's not forget about the obvious muscles in your arms and legs. You need them to be relaxed and to help you conserve energy, because if your body flakes out, your resolve won't be far behind.

Given the endurance levels you're going to need, the exercise routine is very gentle and moderate. This is because, like the rest of the programme, you're looking at cumulative fitness, rather than sporadic and intense bursts of activity. You can start by just moving about more: cycle to the shops, walk an extra bus stop, join an antenatal yoga class. You'd be amazed what a difference building your stamina makes to your labour.

The Exercise Programme

Daily
- Yoga

  This will increase your muscular strength (for pushing and getting into your delivery positions) and flexibility (you'll be amazed where legs and feet end up during birth). Yoga squats can open the pelvis by 30 per cent, which is crucial during labour. You will find the yoga sequence on the following pages. You need to do 20 minutes, first or last thing in the day. However, do bear in mind that yoga is generally not recommended in the first 3 months – it should be gently introduced between 14 and 16 weeks of pregnancy.
- Walking

  Walking is greatly underestimated as a form of exercise but it is one of my favourites. It encourages the baby's head to engage and the 'bounce' of each step can facilitate thinning of the cervix. Don't stroll, walk as briskly as you can without becoming too breathless to speak. You need to do 30 minutes daily, really building up in the last few weeks.

Twice weekly
- Swimming

  This cradles the baby in the bump and helps with foetal positioning. It also takes the weight off the mother's joints – experiencing bouts of weightlessness is a blessing during pregnancy – and is an excellent form of all-over cardiovascular exercise.

  Note: There have recently been concerns about the effects of chlorine during pregnancy, particularly during 'organo-genesis' in the first trimester. There are also links between chlorine and asthma. I recommend swimming in a non-chlorinated pool, such as an ozone-treated pool. If an unchlorinated pool is not available, do not swim more than once a week.

  Caution:
  - Avoid saunas and steamrooms at all stages of your pregnancy.
  - Sunbathing should be limited to only 15 minutes a day.

The Yoga Sequence

Yoga is ideal for the pregnant mother because it encourages suppleness and elasticity. It is also gentle and low-impact so no pressure is placed on the joints. During pregnancy, increased levels of the hormone relaxin circulate around the body. This means that you will feel more limber than usual and it will be easier for you to stretch into the positions, so please take care not to over-stretch yourself. Work within your usual limits of flexibility, even if it feels too 'easy'.

I ask my mothers to perform the following routine every morning when they wake up, but some prefer to do it as a 'wind-down' before going to bed. The sequence was introduced to me by my sister-in-law in India, Jyoti, who used it for her pregnancy and found it wonderfully effective. (Note: A Yoga DVD is available showing a whole routine – see Appendix C, page 314.)

Make sure you are wearing soft, loose clothing that you can move around in freely. Your feet should be bare. Tie your hair back if it is long. If you do not have a yoga mat, a towel is absolutely fine. Keep some squashy cushions, or ideally a beanbag close at hand to relax on.

General guidelines
- When standing, always stand with your feet hip-width apart and avoid locking your knees. You don't need to bend them, but think about keeping your knees 'soft'.
- When you have been lying down and want to return to sitting, roll onto your side and with both hands on the floor, push yourself up. Do not use your stomach and back muscles to pull yourself up.
- Never over-stretch.
- Always do the Introduction and Finale to properly warm up and cool down your muscles.
- If any position feels uncomfortable, abandon it immediately. This is supposed to be a very gentle stretching and breathing programme.
- Try to drink a glass of water about 30 minutes before beginning the routine.
- Relax as and when you need to.

Introduction

1. Stand with your feet hip-width apart, your knees soft. Bring your arms out in front of you, at shoulder height, with your palms touching each other. As you inhale, take your arms out to the sides to form a straight line with your body. Bring them back to the front as you exhale. Repeat 10 times.

2. In the same standing position, drop your arms down to your sides. As you inhale, gently swing your arms forward and up above your head. Carefully swing them back down to your sides as you exhale. Repeat 10 times.

3. Still in the same position, swing your arms in wide circles above your head as you inhale. Cross your arms in front of your chest and arc them out and back down towards your hips as you exhale. Repeat 10 times.

4. Now repeat, this time reversing the direction, bringing the circles inwards. Repeat 10 times.

5. Standing with your arms by your sides, swing your arms outwards and up to your head as you inhale. Bring them back down as you exhale. Repeat 10 times.

Sitting on the floor, legs outstretched

1. Sit on the floor, with your legs outstretched and slightly apart. Your hands should be placed on the floor just at the level of your buttocks, with your palms down and your fingers facing forwards. Rest a little bit of your weight on your arms as you wiggle your toes for a couple of moments. Now flex the feet up and down 5 times.

2. Without lifting your feet off the floor, rotate your ankles inwards, then outwards, 5 times in each direction.

3. Gently lift one straight leg at a time – just about 15cm (6in) off the floor. If this feels a little uncomfortable, lean back further on your arms, or bend your opposite leg at the knee, with the foot flat on the floor. Repeat 5 times on each leg.

4. Sit with your legs slightly further apart and hold your arms out to your sides, at shoulder height. Rotate your waist gently, bringing your left arm forward to touch your right calf (breathing out as you do this). Hold it there for a moment and then, while breathing in, return your arms to their original position and repeat on the other side. Do 5 on each side.

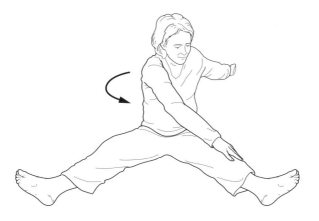

5. Hold your arms out in front of you at shoulder height. Wiggle your fingers for a couple of moments and then flex your hands up and down from the wrist, with your palms facing away from you. Repeat 5 times. Now rotate your hands at the wrist (5 times) and then rotate the whole of your forearm from the elbow (5 times). Do 5 soft bicep curls by touching the top of your shoulders with your fingertips and then flexing and extending your arms. Note: breathing deeply as you perform these exercises is an essential part of yoga as it helps to circulate energy throughout your body.

Relax by placing your hands on the floor behind – fingers facing forward – and resting your weight on your shoulders. Your legs should be relaxed so that your knees roll outwards slightly. Stay in this position for one minute.

Sitting in a cross-legged position

6. Now come into a cross-legged position. Sit forward on your sitting bones (if you aren't quite sure of this position, you may like to place a cushion beneath your hips to tip you forward and straighten your spine – this will automatically bring you onto your sitting bones). Place your hands on your shoulders, with your elbows pointing out, and rotate your arms 15 times in a forward direction and then 15 times in a backwards direction.

7. Inhale and raise your arms above your head, with your palms facing each other. Look up at your fingers and, as you exhale, bring your arms down

and rotate slightly to bring both hands down to your right side, to touch the floor if you can. Inhale again and return your arms above your head. Now exhale and repeat to the left. Repeat slowly 5 times on each side.

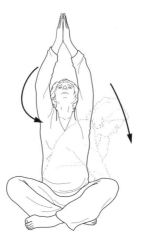

8. With your hands resting on your knees, drop your head and roll forward slightly as you exhale. Return to an upright position as you inhale. Repeat 10 times.

9. Uncurl your legs and bend them in front of you in a diamond shape. With your hands on your ankles pull forward gently as you exhale. Relax up as you inhale. Repeat 10 times.

10. Pranayama (Breathing Sequence). Place your right hand on your right knee. Now take your left hand and, with your palm facing you, curl in the middle three fingers so that your thumb and little finger remain outstretched. Bring your hand to your face and place your thumb on your left nostril, closing it. Inhale deeply through the right nostril. When you are ready to exhale, close your right nostril with your ring finger, lift your thumb off the left nostril and exhale through it. Inhale again, this time through your left nostril and then exhale by placing your thumb over your left nostril and releasing your ring finger off the right side. Exhale. Repeat each pranayam separately between 10 and 20 times. Breathe very slowly and deeply. Return your hand to your lap and rest for 2–3 regular breaths between each set of this breathing sequence.

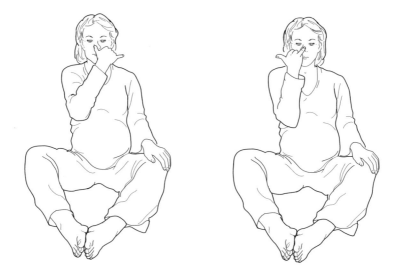

11. Change your position so that you come to sit on your heels. If your bump is very big, position your thighs wide apart. Clasp your hands behind your back and, as you exhale, gently roll forward as far as you can. Hold for a moment, then return to an upright position as you inhale. Repeat 5 times.

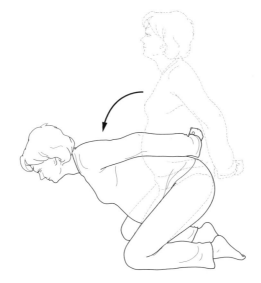

12. Cradle your arms so that each hand nestles in the crook of the opposite elbow. Inhale, with your head bowed, and as you exhale, lean forward, extending your arms and placing your hands on your calves or ankles. Hold the pose for a moment then inhale and return to the cradle position. Repeat 5 times.

Relax by letting your head drop forward slightly; bring your hands to rest on your knees. Relax for 1 minute.

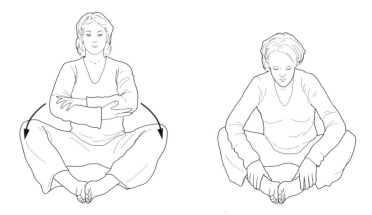

Lying down – leg exercises

If you are more than 20 weeks pregnant, you may find lying on your back uncomfortable – in this case, recline on some cushions or a beanbag, which will keep you at a certain angle.

13. Bend your left leg, placing the foot flat on the floor. Slowly rotate your right leg so that the knee points outwards and raise the right leg to 45 degrees. Return it to the floor and repeat on the other side. Do this 5 times with each leg.

14. With your legs outstretched and your arms by your side, slowly bend your left leg, bringing your foot flat on the floor as close as possible to your bottom. Return it to the floor and repeat on the other side. Repeat 5 times on each leg.

Relax by lying back with your legs relaxed (knees pointing outwards) and your palms facing up. Stay there for 2 minutes.

15. Return to a sitting position, with one leg outstretched and the other bent, with the foot resting alongside the opposite knee and cradling both arms in front of the waist. As you exhale, lean forward and bring your hands onto the calf of the bent leg. Hold for a moment then inhale and return to an upright position. Repeat on the other side. Repeat 5 times.

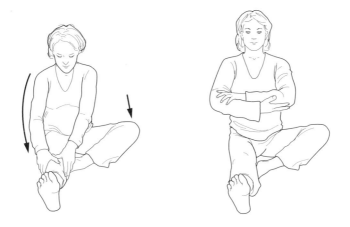

Finale

16. Stand up with your feet hip-width apart and your arms stretched out in front of you at shoulder height. Exhale and gently bend your knees, keeping your back straight and your heels on the floor. Inhale and stand up straight again. Repeat 5 times.

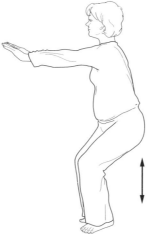

Wind-down

17. Stand with your feet hip-width apart, your knees soft. Bring your arms out in front of you, at shoulder height. As you inhale, expand your arms out to the side. Bring them back to the front as you exhale. Repeat 10 times.

18. Standing, drop your arms down to your sides. As you inhale, gently swing your arms forward and up above your head. Carefully swing them back down as you exhale. Repeat 10 times.

19. Now swing your arms in wide circles, crossing in front of your chest and arcing out and back down towards your hips. Repeat 10 times.

20. Repeat the exercise, this time reversing the direction, bringing the circles inwards. Repeat 10 times.

21. Standing with your arms by your sides, swing your arms outwards and up to your head as you inhale. Bring them back down as you exhale. Repeat 5 times.

22. Lie down on your left-hand side as comfortably as possible, stretching yourself out. Rest deeply for at least 5–10 minutes.

Adding a mantra

If you wish to add sound therapy to your yoga practice, chanting mantras can be very useful. A mantra is a sound sequence that is repeated over and over again. Some yogis chant mantras for hours and even days on end, but for the average mother even 10 minutes of chanting creates a sense of peace and harmony.

Simply sit in a comfortable position and repeat your chosen mantra in a lilting voice over and over again for as long as you can. This can be deeply relaxing and your baby is also gently massaged by the vibrations of the mantra. The following mantra in Sanskrit is simple and calming.

OM NAMA SHIVA

(TRANSLATION: I ACKNOWLEDGE THAT I AM PART OF THE DIVINE SOURCE)

On occasion when I have treated an agitated mother, or indeed a stressed woman who is trying to conceive, I have chanted this with them for at least 30 minutes as I administered reflexology or Creative Healing and have noticed a deep sense of peace descending on them.

As an alternative, try the Gayatri Mantra, referred to as the supreme mantra by the sages. Again, it is chanted in Sanskrit (the translation is given below the mantra):

OM BUR BURVASVAHA

TAT SAVITUR VARENGYAM

BHARGO DEVASYA DHIMAHI

DIHYO YONAH PRACHODAYAT

OM SHANTI, SHANTI, SHANTI

LORD OF THE THREE WORLDS

YOU ARE THE ULTIMATE TRUTH

SHINE YOUR LIGHT ON ME

AND GUIDE MY INTELLECT

PEACE, PEACE, PEACE

If you do not wish to repeat a mantra yourself, you could try to obtain a pre-recorded tape or CD of a mantra and play it in the background as you perform your yoga. (Try alternative bookshops, health food stores and shops selling Eastern or so-called 'new-age' products. We also have a CD with the above Mantras – see Appendix C, page 314.)

Exercises for Labour

There are many exercises you can do during labour to reduce your discomfort, particularly if the baby is in an awkward position. I have placed them here, rather than in the Labour section, so that you may practise them in advance. These are demonstrated on the Jeyarani *Yoga for Pregnancy* DVD – see Appendix C, page 314.)

Figure of eight

Stand with your legs shoulder-width apart and, with your legs slightly bent, rotate your hips in a figure of eight. This helps cradle the baby in to the front of the bump, reducing pressure on the spine. Repeat as often as you want, changing direction sporadically.

The camel walk

This is like doing the 'sand dance' only you don't have to wear a fez! Walk forward with an exaggerated walk, lifting your legs high up like you're stepping over some logs. At the same time tip your pelvis and belly backwards and forwards in an up and down circular motion. Some mothers find it helps to think of their pelvis as a scoop. This is very funny to do and watch – but it is also effective in reducing lower back pain.

Elephant walk

Walk forward with giant steps but this time, with every step, rotate your lifted knee outwards as far as you can (abducting your thigh to the side) and then, while still keeping your trunk facing forward, set your foot down on the ground. You will notice that you cannot walk in a straight line but move around the room in a zig-zag line. This helps to increase the diameter of your pelvis.

The Charlie Chaplin walk

You have seen Charlie Chaplin walk in the old black and white movies. Now it's time to imitate him! Walk forwards, taking small steps, with your feet pointing outwards, loose hips and a sloppy gait. This will loosen your pelvic ligaments and open the pelvis just that little bit further.

I'm indebted to Dr Françoise Freedman, anthropologist and originator of Birthlight yoga, for introducing me to the funny walks and the use of the breath while performing the vaginal stretch technique.

Crawling on all fours

This is very good for optimal foetal positioning. It simply involves crawling around the room like a baby on all fours for a couple of minutes at a time. I especially recommend this exercise after 32 weeks when the baby begins to have less room to move about, and the position the baby settles in becomes more important.

You should also be aware of the possible positions you will assume when you are in labour. See 'Positions in labour' on page 192. Yoga will help you achieve these positions but where possible you should also practise them.

Mental Preparation

The Mind as Muscle

So far, we have seen how diet and physical therapies can help train the uterus for birth fitness, clearing it of toxins and leaving it clean, unobstructed and strong for labour. In principle, the mental preparation element of the programme requires just such the same commitment – cleansing, toning and exercising the mind like a muscle. But for many of my mothers, this is the hardest part of the programme. A body can be cleared of toxins, stresses and anxieties far more easily than the mind. The laying of hands onto flesh is instant balm, but it takes more than cuddles and massage to console and encourage the mind, especially in our western culture where the media and, let's be honest, our family and friends regale us with birth horror stories.

It's little wonder that we face labour with trepidation and fear, when shocking stories are passed down as fact, and social conditioning packages the birth process as a desperate struggle. Quite simply, we're never given the opportunity to see that birth can be a gentle, relaxed, comfortable process, where labour is a dance between the mother and her baby – both bodies in step with each other, following the rhythms of contractions. The body instinctively knows what to do. It's the fear and anxiety lodged in our minds that gets in the way and causes our bodies to tense up. However, by reconditioning your attitudes towards birth, you can learn not only how to control the level of pain you feel but to use simple mental exercises – like visualizations and 'safe places' – that can act like anaesthetics. You simply have to view your mind, not as a nebulous mental space, but as another muscle in your body that you can flex, tone and control.

The Power of Positive Suggestion

Fear is one of the greatest barriers to having a gentle birth because it releases the 'fight or flight' hormone, adrenalin. This has a constrictive effect on the body, causing tightening of the muscles and even going so far as to stop the cervix from opening and the uterus from contracting efficiently. The mental element of the programme teaches you to eliminate fear and anxiety through the following means:

1. Deep muscle relaxation – this physical exercise is a necessary precursor to the mental exercises, removing all physical resistance and letting the body go through the mechanics of labour efficiently and quickly, while the mind escapes.
2. Self-hypnosis – this engenders a positive mental attitude towards birth, making you feel that it is something you can achieve naturally, hence you feel more in control of the labour process.
3. Safe places – the ability to take your mind away to a safe place that you can visualize is a powerful coping tool for managing the pain of contractions.
4. Visualization – by using this technique you can learn what to expect of your body both during pregnancy and labour, which reduces the fear of the unknown.
5. Birth rehearsals – these prepare you for meeting your baby and hasten your progress through labour.

The Science of Self-hypnosis

Hypnosis is a naturally occurring state of intense concentration coupled with deep relaxation.

PROFESSOR DAVID SPIEGEL, STANFORD UNIVERSITY

The success of self-hypnosis in enabling the mind to control the body has been proven in numerous fields – from stress management and psychotherapy to giving up smoking and curing phobias – and much of the current research has moved on to how hypnosis can control the levels of pain we feel. During hypnosis there is increased blood flow in the part of the brain that is associated with dreams – this capacity has been evaluated by a technique called Positron Emission Tomography, which detects increased blood flow. During hypnosis your brain exhibits alpha waves and these automatically result in the release of endorphins, the body's natural painkillers – just what you want when you're in labour. In labour, alpha waves also increase the release of the hormone oxytocin – thereby progressing labour – and help your baby's placenta release hormones that cause the muscles within your pelvis to become soft, open, relaxed and slippery – perfect conditions for a gentle birth.

Self-doubt – Your Biggest Obstacle

So, do you think you can do it? If your immediate response is 'no', then what you have to tackle and overcome is not chemistry, but scepticism. It's the single, biggest obstacle many of my mothers face in this section of the programme. Following a diet and exercise regime is a part of modern life for many women the world over, so practising one while pregnant isn't an issue, but the prospect of meditation and self-hypnosis intimidates a lot of women who feel it's not something they can do, or worse, want to do.

Hypnosis has been used obstetrically since the 1830s, when it was deployed as an anaesthetic towards the end of labour, but it fell out of favour when showgrounds adopted it as a form of entertainment and it quickly became associated with quackery. Ever since then, stage hypnosis has done a lot of damage to its therapeutic reputation, implying that people are subject to the power of the hypnotist and can be forced into actions against their will. This is not the case. You cannot hypnotize someone to do something they really don't want to do, or make them do something that goes against their moral code or ethics. Hypnosis can only reinforce something you already want to do.

With regard to how to do it – well you already know. Self-hypnosis is simply a technical term for something that we all do all the time – day-dreaming is another, gentler term for it. Several times a day you may glide into a deeply relaxed daydream state without even noticing. So there's no challenge in it – slipping into a hypnotic state is something you've been doing your whole life. My aim is simply to show you how to harness it at will to become a conscious, rather than subconscious, tool.

The secret is conditioning, conditioning, conditioning. If you make something normal to you, it will become instinctive. The more you train your body and mind before the labour, the more easily your body will respond when you need it to. I strongly encourage my mothers to listen to the self-hypnosis audiotape (you can either use the pre-recorded tape available from Jeyarani or record your own) every day after 20 weeks, and ideally before then. Starting up just a few weeks before the birth places so much more pressure on the body and mind. If it can become a part of your daily routine early on in your pregnancy – and many of my mothers welcome the tape as a good excuse for 'me time' indulgence anyway – you can really relax in the knowledge that you're giving yourself the training time you need for self-hypnosis to become an automatic reflex. Another common misconception about hypnosis is that it induces a catatonic state. In fact, you remain aware but simply deeply relaxed. Also, because you will be using self-hypnosis, you can lighten or deepen your level of hypnosis according to your needs – something that is particularly valuable during the birth process when you may want to move around.

Many of my mothers are nervous that while they can induce a self-hypnotic state at home or at one of my classes, they will be unable to do it during labour, due to the discomfort of contractions 'pulling' them out of their relaxed state. This is a very common concern and something that you can dismiss if you've put in the practice. Trust in yourself. I have literally hundreds of letters from mothers who testify their amazement at how easy it was to enter and remain in varying degrees of hypnosis throughout their labours (even while moving about), using visualization to manage the peak of the contractions and then slipping back into a deeper state of hypnosis between tightenings.

Hypnosis can also make time pass more quickly. Whenever I ask the mothers in my classes to estimate how long they have been in a state of hypnosis, estimates vary from 10–20 minutes, when in fact the elapsed time is usually 45 minutes.

When body and mind are synchronized in relaxation, birthing is essentially easy to manage – as it is for other mammals. Through self-hypnosis, you can move into a state of deep muscle relaxation and enable the body to become highly elastic, mobile and flexible for an efficient, short and gentle birth. So let's learn how.

Tip: The secrets of cervical dilatation

The quickest way to 10cm is through Deep Muscle Relaxation, which improves blood flow to the whole body, particularly the cervix and uterus. Visualizations of the pelvis opening, widening, warming and loosening compound those effects.

Birth Story: Visualizing a thin cervix – Andrea

My due date wasn't for another five days, so although I had visualized the baby's head dropping deep into my pelvis, I didn't recognize the start of my proper contractions. I felt energized at work all day, not bothering to finish at lunchtime as usual. Experiencing what I thought were just Braxton-Hicks, I drove an hour through the London traffic to spend an evening with my best friend. We laughed about the curry she cooked sending me into early labour – little did we know how right we were!

Driving home, I still perceived the period-like pains as Braxton-Hicks so I stopped off at a local restaurant for some tea and a chat with my brother-in-law for an hour or so.

On climbing into bed at midnight, I tried to settle, but although with the use of my safe place I had nodded off, the strength of my contractions woke me. By 1.30am, I realized this must be the real thing and promptly ran a bath. At about 2am, I had a show and felt very excited as I realized this was definitely 'it.'

From 3am or so, back in bed and going to my safe place, I dozed in and out of sleep, giving my husband's hand a squeeze every time I experienced a contraction. At 5am, Nigel announced that I had had seven contractions, five minutes apart, and we ought to ring the midwives.

I was having a home birth, so it was great not to have to get dressed and go out into the cold. The first midwife arrived at 6am and examined me. She was amazed (considering this was my first child) as I was already 3cm dilated and she exclaimed 'my goodness, your cervix is so thin'. Of course it was – I had spent the last 13 weeks telling it to be thin.

My contractions were coming at varying intervals, sometimes three to four minutes apart, sometimes seven or eight. After another bath, they sped up slightly and when the second midwife arrived at 7.30am, I was 7cm dilated.

I was not expecting so much discomfort in my back, but Nigel and the midwives continually massaged it as I, positioned on all fours on the bed, buried my head in the pillows in a trance-like state between contractions, off in my safe place.

When the contractions were every three minutes or so, I asked for the gas and air. It did absolutely nothing to help ease the worst of the contractions but it did give me something to bite on and squeeze.

I wasn't able to fully maintain my hypnotic state during the peak of the contraction, but being in my safe place between them helped to conserve my energy and allowed me to focus on the next one. I told myself each contraction brought my baby closer to me and, the stronger they were, the better they were doing their job. I thought of each contraction as a wave crashing onto a beach. As the waves crashed, there was tremendous force, but the beautiful sensation of the water flowing away and seeping back out to sea made it all worthwhile. As each one ebbed away, I felt an amazing sense of peace, and almost euphoria.

It was then my waters broke. It was 8.20am and I was fully dilated. I started to push, but hadn't expected it to be such an effort. It took a few contractions before I realized I had to hold the push to prevent the baby's head from slipping back in. Two or three contractions later, I braced against Nigel, the baby slipped out and I heard someone say 'It's a girl.' Baby Jade was born at 8.30am, just three and a half hours after I started regularly contracting. Weighing 7lb 2oz, she was a perfect size to get through my pelvis.

I am convinced that the ease of the birth is due to my sticking to all the advice given in the programme. It is essential to stick to the dietary advice. It may be restrictive, but it's not prohibitive and it was well worth it for the energy and sense of well-being it gave me. Throughout my pregnancy, I was constantly congratulated on looking so well and healthy. In spite of my fears, the visualization and self-hypnosis classes did work – even my husband believed it once he heard the midwife comment on the thinness of my cervix!

My advice to anyone is to heed all the instructions in the programme and follow them. If you really believe it, it will be the birth you really want and deserve.

Deep Muscle Relaxation and Self-hypnosis – Getting Started

Over the rest of this chapter you will find the transcripts for some deep muscle relaxation, self-hypnosis and visualization exercises. I have written them out here as an introduction to the images and vocabulary that are typical of these mental techniques and so that you may practise as and when you like. Read through this chapter and then, if you would like to, record all the transcripts onto a cassette tape so that you can listen to them on a regular basis. How you make up these tapes is up to you. You may like to tape the Self-hypnosis Script (pages 95–9) on side A of the tape, and listen to this side often until you feel that you can switch off very quickly. On the other side of the tape, record the Visualization Script (the Secret Garden on pages 107–9, and/or the Lift on page 110). After this, on the same side of the tape, you may like to record the Pre-programming for Labour Script (pages 112–16). Alternatively you can make tapes with your own combination of scripts. Remember that all these mental exercises (self-hypnosis, visualizations, safe places and labour rehearsal) are interlinked. For example, you can't move into self-hypnosis if the body is not in a state of deep relaxation, and the powerful and positive suggestions made to you in the labour visualization will have no impact if you are not in a hypnotic state. For this reason until you are sufficiently efficient at self-hypnosis, always listen to side A of your tape before listening to the visualizations etc on the other side. Once you can easily switch off you can listen to the scripts on side B straight away. For those readers who would like more direct help, I have produced some audio tapes featuring deep muscle relaxation and self-hypnosis techniques and various visualizations – these are available from my clinic. Please refer to Appendix C, pages 313–14 at the back of the book for further details. For simplicity's sake, in this book I shall refer to your tape and the Jeyarani tape as the 'self-hypnosis tape'.

Now let's look at the practicalities of self-hypnosis. Relaxation and self-hypnosis is done with the eyes closed, because when they are shut, your brain automatically changes its electrical wave pattern to alpha waves, a highly receptive mode. I like to induce deep muscle relaxation through the technique of tensing and then loosening each set of muscles in the body. We will work upwards from the feet, all the way to the top of the head. As you do this, you will notice that you are gradually becoming more and more relaxed, so that by the time we reach your facial muscles, you will be so relaxed that you're just a step away from hypnosis.

When you first begin practising the following exercise, lie down or sit back in a quiet, preferably darkened, room where you can't hear the telephone. (Once you become accustomed to it, you will be able to induce deep relaxation virtually anywhere.)

If you don't want to record the following transcript onto a tape, you can ask your partner or birthing partner – someone with whom you have implicit trust and confidence – to read the following transcript to you. Whether recording the script or simply reading it, the speaker should soften their voice and slow down their speech to help encourage relaxation.

Self-hypnosis Script

Close your eyes and breathe deeply for a minute. Take three deep breaths and with each exhalation tell yourself 'I'm going into hypnosis now'. From this point onward, these words will act as an instant trigger to your body to relax, automatically putting you in a receptive mode.

With your eyelids closed, allow your inner eye to scan the muscles on the inside of your body, starting from your feet and moving upwards through your legs, thighs, hips, lower back, upper back, neck, and shoulders. Now let go of your attention on your muscles, let your eyelids open and fix your gaze on an imaginary spot directly overhead. You will notice as I count from 1 to 10, your eyelids become heavier and heavier; so heavy that on the count of ten you will allow your eyelids to come to lie one against the other in deep relaxation.

So here we go: one, two, three, four – getting dreamier and sleepier; five, six, seven, eight – going deeper and deeper; nine and ten, very deeply relaxed as you allow your body to gently float into total muscle relaxation, as I talk you through a guided visualization.

Imagine that the tiny muscles in your eyelids have become very soft and silky as they lie closed in deep relaxation. Now allow that same relaxation to flow down from your eyelids, down your face, neck and shoulders, down your whole body, right to the very tips of your toes. Allow this relaxation to flow rhythmically down your body like waves that flow down from the top of your head to the tips of your toes. With every breath you take, you feel the soft sensation of relaxation flowing down your whole body, and with every breath you take you become more and more relaxed and all the muscles in your body begin to feel like soft, velvety silk.

Now I would like you to take your attention to the muscles around your hips and pelvis. This is a very important area; during pregnancy, the pelvic floor muscle supports your uterus, within which your baby grows. The pelvic floor looks like a bowl of muscle that supports your beautiful uterus. On either side of the muscle, are networks of blood vessels, lymphatics and nerves that are all embedded in connective tissue and fatty tissue.

I now invite you to exercise the pelvic floor by contracting your hips and buttocks – feel the squeeze within your pelvis. Now relax and let go and feel how the circulation of this area has speeded up. Visualize that the extra tissue fluid from the pelvis has been squeezed out and pumped back through the lymphatic system to the kidneys, leaving the hips and pelvis feeling light and clear. Take a deep breath in – and out.

Now take your attention to the whole of your back. Your vertebral column stretches all the way up from your tiny tail bones, up through your sacrum or back bone, lower back, upper back and neck. The first vertebrae on the top of your spine articulates with the base of your skull, helping you to stand upright. On either side of the spinal column are rows of strong muscles called the para-vertebral muscles, which are like pillars supporting your spine on either side. There are also small muscles between each vertebra that give your spine mobility in several directions. There are other curvaceous muscles in your back, which give your back a beautiful shape.

I'd like you now to squeeze all those muscles and feel your spine arch forwards and your head pull back. Now let go and imagine the disc spaces at the base of your spine, and encourage them to plump up for better circulation of fluids in the body. Feel how the spinal column has elongated and becomes even more comfortable as the nerves are freed up; feel the relaxation flow all the way round the chest cage, thighs, tops of thighs to tips of your toes – as every part of the body is touched by this new invigorated blood flow.

Now, see the flat muscles at the front of the tummy, muscles which hold the baby in place in the abdominal cavity. See the vertical muscles from the sternum to the pubis, give them a nice squeeze, and let go. Allow the abdomen to feel softer and relaxed. This gives the baby the sense of what it's like to have space to move and be free, in preparation for life outside the womb.

Now take your attention to the triangular muscles of your neck and shoulders, which stretch from the tip of your earlobes down to the tips of your shoulders. The outer muscle within your neck is called the trapezius and the deeper muscles are called the scalene muscles. It is of vital importance for the health of your whole body to focus on relaxing your neck muscles. So contract them, slowly squeezing them by lifting the tips of your shoulders right up to your ears; hold them there for a few seconds and then drop them down suddenly. Imagine that your shoulders are falling away from the tips of your earlobes, right down towards your waist. Imagine an inner hand is gently strumming the muscles of your neck, taking away all tension and smoothing out the knots. Take another deep breath – in and out – as you go deeper and deeper into total muscle relaxation.

Tighten your arm muscles and then relax. Every time you squeeze the arms and then let them drop down, you double the depth of relaxation. Take your shoulders into a shrug and then let go.

Finally, allow all the muscles in your face to scrunch up, squeezing your eyes shut and making all the muscles contract as much as you can. And now relax and let go. You feel a warm flush underneath the skin of your face as fresh blood flows in underneath your cheeks.

Now open your eyes, look straight ahead, and then let them shut again. Take three more deep breaths into the lowest part of your abdomen. Now imagine that you are lying on a sandy beach in the shade of a palm tree, and you're looking at a beautiful blue lagoon. As you gaze at the water, the gently lapping waves seem to keep pace with your breath. A wonderful cool breeze comes in and beautifully strokes your skin. You lie there admiring the peace and tranquillity of the lagoon. You feel so relaxed throughout your body that you don't want to twitch even a single muscle.

With your inner eye, imagine moving into the water and floating on your back, allowing the water to support you completely. You feel the warmth of the water lapping all over you and you go deeper and deeper into muscle relaxation. The warm tropical water seems to take away all your tension and tiredness, and you sigh deeply as you fall deeper and deeper into total muscle relaxation. You imagine that someone who cares for you is standing beside you gently holding your shoulders and rocking you to sleep; and you sleep deeply, very deeply. You are more relaxed than ever before. You feel very safe and looked after.

From now on, whenever you want to relax, every time your eyelids shut and you take three deep breaths into the lowest part of your abdomen, you will be completely and totally relaxed in every muscle fibre of your body. In the twinkling of an eye, you will allow all your body rhythms to wind down to their baseline levels of deep rest and relaxation. Every breath you take goes down deep into the pelvis, making it looser and wider, and making it easier for the baby to drift down further into it – and then out. When you are in labour, you may like to take three deep breaths with every contraction to deepen the relaxation and aid this process.

Now, very slowly and gradually, I'd like you to come back to full awareness of the room around you, feeling tingly all over; feeling mentally refreshed and rejuvenated.'

When you have become familiar with the content of this script, you will no longer be dependent upon the tape or the voice of your partner to ease you into deep muscle relaxation and self-hypnosis. Wherever you are, all you will have to do is to find a comfortable position, sitting or lying down, let your eyelids close, take three deep breaths into the lowest part of your abdomen and say 'I'm going into self-hypnosis now'. Try to test yourself at various points throughout the day in different locations – on the bus, at your desk, in the bath. Don't worry if it takes a short while for you to really notice a reaction. The subconscious mind has been likened to that of a four-year old, so repetition is key. Keep practising, the body needs time to learn the response.

Once you have taken yourself into self-hypnosis, you then breathe normally and invite your mind to take you to your safe place, where only good things can happen to you. (We will be looking at how you can construct and use your 'safe place' in the Visualization section on page 106). At this point you then allow your mind to rehearse the natural events that will happen in a smooth and easy sequence on the expected day of your delivery (this visualization is featured on page 111).

As a result of practising this over and over again, on the day you go into labour you will automatically go into self-hypnosis, you will be calm and sure of yourself, and you will be able to relax all the muscles in your body both during and between contractions. The only muscles that will have to act will be the automatic muscles in your body – your heart, your respiratory muscles and the spontaneous muscle action of your uterus.

When you practise deep self-hypnosis from the very first uterine contraction, you can programme every subsequent contraction to feel twice as comfortable as the previous one. I have noted that those mothers who really apply themselves to the self-hypnosis programme often report to me that they felt most comfortable just as the baby was being born and that they really enjoyed the sensation of the baby coming out of their body.

Birth story: Countering pain with hypnotherapy – Jane, a GP

I had not been planning anything revolutionary for the birth of my first child. It was going to be a managed hospital delivery, with plenty of pain relief. The notion of alternatives like waterbirths hadn't entered my head, but then, by chance, I met Dr Motha, who invited me to attend her classes.

I have to confess that I was sceptical about whether hypnotherapy could really work in easing labour and reducing pain, but I was prepared to have a go at it. I went once a week, and then every other week towards the end of the pregnancy.

After a few sessions it was quite easy to get the hang of, and we had to go home and practise with the help of our partners. Although it appeared to work in our sessions with Dr Motha, I was still unconvinced it would work for me in labour.

I know it sounds silly for a doctor to say, but I'm a wimp when it comes to pain. I had seen a lot of pain and suffering experienced by women in labour and the thought of having to go through such an ordeal really frightened me. I couldn't see how mind over matter could be better than pethidine and entonox. Nonetheless, lying on a sun-drenched Greek beach and the sensation of floating on air were my chosen alternatives.

So when my waters broke at 2.30am, one morning, I cast myself off to my Greek island and experienced very little pain. I couldn't believe how well it was working. When I should have been feeling

---

pain at the height of each contraction, there was none. I kept thinking this couldn't last, but it did.

I called Dr Motha who said she would come round to examine me. By then I was experiencing pain down the sides of my legs and beginning to think I was a failure and hadn't done the hypno-therapy properly. Looking back, I think the discomfort must have been caused by the way the baby was lying – it must have been touching a nerve.

When Gowri arrived and examined me, she said I was almost fully dilated. I was flabbergasted, particularly as this was my first baby. Three and a quarter hours after starting labour, my son Oscar was born. The delivery was calm and stress-free, and my blood pressure was low. My pulse was only 64, when it should have been much higher.

Father's tip: Deepening hypnosis

Let the mother settle into self-hypnosis, then reach out and gently, using the tip of your index finger, stroke her face from the hairline in the centre of her fore-head straight down to the tip of her nose. Repeat this a few times. As you stroke her tell her, 'You are going deeper and deeper into self-hypnosis.'

Now open your hands so that they are flat, place them on her shoulders and gently push down, softly saying 'you are going deeper into relaxation.' You are trying to reinforce the sense of her limbs feeling heavy and weighted. Switch between stroking her face and gently stroking down her arms. As you do so whisper encouragement such as 'You are doing so well', 'Your pelvis is wide and open', 'I'm so proud of you', 'Every breath you take is making you more and more relaxed'.

Remember to use only supportive and positive language.

This is a very bonding exercise and if you practise a lot before the birth it will help to increase your partner's level of self-hypnosis and relaxation. The more you practise this exercise, the quicker you can access this tool during labour. Your touch will release endorphins for the mother and make her feel safe. It reaffirms the trust between you and lets the mother know you are looking after her and the baby. This really can be a vital resource in helping the mother stay in emotional control, but you must practise as much as possible before the labour begins, in order for her relaxation response to your touch to become automatic.

Note: Some mothers find that when they go into labour, they do not want to be touched at all. This is OK and very common. Don't be hurt if your partner doesn't want to be touched by you but would prefer to retreat inside herself. You can still support her by protecting her environment – keeping the lights low, minimizing noise and disturbances, and stopping people barging into the room and speaking loudly to her.

Signs of a good, deep hypnosis

- Muscle twitching – a neuro-muscular response. As your body enters a deep hypnotic state, the muscles may twitch because the nerve supply to them suddenly gets very high levels of oxygen, due to the increase in size of the blood vessels that supply the brain and all the nerves of the body.
- Redness in the whites of the eyes. As described above, when we fully relax dilatation of the blood vessels occurs. The capillaries in the whites of the eyes are the only place in the body where we can actually see this dilatation occurring.
- Increased need to swallow. This is due to increased salivation caused by dilation of your salivary ducts.
- A feeling of warmth encroaching over your body due to the increased capillary dilatation.
- Your body feels incredibly wide or your body outline feels blurred.
- You may experience pins and needles in your fingers and toes as the muscles fully relax and there is increased blood supply to nerves.

Father's Tip: How to test for deep muscle relaxation – the arm drop

When your partner is in deep relaxation, gently lift one of her arms by the thumb about 20cm (8in) up into the air. Gently rock the arm for about a minute while you quietly make suggestions to her that her whole body is becoming as soft and loose as the arm that you are holding. Then whisper the suggestion that as you drop her arm to her lap, she will double the relaxation in her whole body, including her pelvis. Then, quite suddenly and without prior warning, drop her arm onto her lap. If she is truly relaxed, her arm will fall suddenly and heavily to her side. If she is not deeply relaxed, the arm will hover by itself in the air, or drop in a controlled manner to her lap. It is essential to get the confidence of the mother so that she can let go of her mind and detach from all muscle tension. This comes with practise and mutual trust in each other, as well as trust in the benefits of self-hypnosis for managing labour.

Birth Story: Holding on to fear – Sally

I started pre-labour at 1am with diarrhoea and crampy pains. I didn't know it was pre-labour, I really believed it was just diarrhoea, which seems ridiculous now, after all that I had read about diarrhoea being a sign of pre-labour!

I slept until about 8am after emptying my bowels during the night several times. I still had crampy feelings in the morning, like slight period pains, but continued the day as normal. I went shopping and had lunch at a restaurant.

By about 2pm, the cramps were coming and going, but were still not uncomfortable, though by this time I had realized this was probably the beginning of labour. I went home and lay down at 3.30pm for half an hour and as I got up my waters broke – it wasn't a big gush as I had thought it would be, just about a cupful of water.

I then saw that the mucus plug had come away when I went to the toilet and the water coming out had some white specks in it, which the midwives told me was vernix from the baby. At that point the contractions started properly – rather than just the earlier period-type pain – and from then on, they felt quite strong, coming at about 10-minute intervals. This was now about 4pm. so I called the hospital and was told to wait at home, have a bath and to call them at 7pm So I put on some music and had a bath, which I found comforting.

When I went into hospital at 7pm, the contractions felt very intense with a lot of pressure on my back passage almost from the beginning. It was this feeling that was taking the breath out of me and I found it the most difficult part of the pain management. My contractions were coming every 2–3 minutes and when the midwife examined me, I was 4cm dilated.

Because of the self-hypnosis techniques I had learnt in the classes, time seemed to go by in a dream. The lights were dimmed and I automatically mentally retreated into another place once my contractions started and it continued that way throughout the labour. I concentrated on one contraction at a time, without thinking about the next hour or next minute. I did it without thinking – it just seemed to be the easiest way to deal with everything.

My partner was with me throughout the whole labour and I used him to lean on during the contractions, which was helpful. He barely spoke either, except to gee me along at the height of contractions. At one point though, while I was in the pool, I thought there was a change in the mood of the room and I thought it was because my partner was feeling impatient and a bit concerned, so I asked him to leave for a while and to go for a walk. When I asked him afterwards if he had been feeling anxious at that point, he said he had not, so I don't know what the change in atmosphere was – maybe I just became more aware of his presence and needed to withdraw again.

During the labour, I thought to myself 'this is brutal' but it was as if I was just observing what my body was doing. It was not so much a feeling of pain, but the physicality of it, actually feeling my body being taken over by the contractions, the forces of nature doing their most primal raw job of opening my body to give birth.

After 3 hours of standing, walking and moving my hips in a figure of eight movement, which helped, I asked if I could get into the birthing pool. This was about 10pm. As soon as I got into the pool, the next contraction was totally different to the ones before and I felt like a fish flopping itself out onto dry land, I literally almost did. It took me completely by surprise – this must have been the beginning of the second stage but I was so taken aback, I called the midwife in and asked if it was normal. It was from this point that my body really seemed to take over. The feeling of the contractions pushing the uterus down from the top was very powerful, and it was amazing to be aware of my body completely taking over and doing its thing!

I actually didn't let go as much as I should have; I held on to a little bit of fear and surprise, which meant that I was not breathing with the contractions very well, so I felt winded. Looking back, it was at this point that I could have really gone with it all and breathed with it and helped my body in its labour efforts, but I did fight against it a little, which made it a bit harder. I came out of the pool and squatted to give birth to my daughter, Ella.

At the last stages there was some concern because the monitor was showing that her heart rate was slowing down and not recovering quickly after each contraction. The midwife was concerned and she called on an obstetrician to assess the situation. But I wasn't worried because I saw that Ella's heart rate recovered after each contraction when I breathed into each contraction and didn't fight it. I watched this happen on the monitor that was monitoring Ella's heart, and I knew it was to do with my breathing. I concentrated on my breath and eventually, after a lot of pushing, she came out at 1.21am. It was a wonderful relief. My partner held Ella on his chest until I brought her onto the bed to feed her.

❀ Visualizations

To do a visualization you must be deeply relaxed and be in a state of self-hypnosis (so that your mind is receptive to positive thoughts). You will then be ready to move through a visualization.

Your Safe Place – Managing Contractions and Reducing Pain

Visualization of a retreat, or 'safe place', is going to be your best tool for managing contractions. It's a mental distraction technique that reduces the amount of pain the brain registers and allows your body to work efficiently. The brain may be limited to your body, but your mind is not. It spans the universe and can fly away from a situation, be playful, consoling, or switched off.

To build a picture of an emotional retreat, I start by asking the mother to imagine a place where she remembers feeling truly relaxed, totally unhurried and untroubled. For many, this is a holiday memory – stretched out on a sandy beach at sunset, lying under a tree in a garden, swinging in a hammock, dozing on a gently rocking boat. But choose whatever you like – it doesn't need to be a memory. You may just respond to one of the ideas above. I find a lot of mothers like to think of a garden, with steps leading down to ever-deeper levels of comfort and safety. The important thing is that it's somewhere you like to think about, that you can clearly visualize, and somewhere that you'll want to keep coming back to.

Then fill in the gaps of your dreamscape – what time of day is it? Who else is there, or are you alone? How does the sun feel on your tummy? Can you feel your hair tickling your neck in the breeze? Is there a distant hum of background noise or is everything silent? Try imagining your safe place using all your five senses: sight, touch, smell, taste and sound. It might seem funny to say that a place has a taste but if you're by the sea you may be able to taste salt in the air, or some people say they can taste the essence of flowers – try it, you might surprise yourself. The more details you can build up of your safe place the better.

Build up your picture, and then come back to it again and again. Get to know it well and add new details as you go along. If you would like to share every detail of your safe place with your partner. Even if you would prefer to keep the details of your safe place to yourself, choose some trigger words that instantly conjur up the retreat and share these with your partner. The father can play a crucial role in assisting visualization during labour, as he can observe and help the mother retreat to her safe place when she needs to, helping her to stay in control.

If you wish you can use the following visualization as your safe place, or simply use it as an example to help you build up your own. You can get your partner to read it to you until you become familiar with it, or you can record it yourself.

Secret Garden Visualization Script
As I count from one to five, let your eyelids shut and visualize a secret garden. Imagine there are five steps leading down to it and as we slowly descend, it will feel even more inviting than before. So here we go. One, it feels deep and cool; two, the warm sun is shining all over your body as you notice how drowsy you are; three, you feel your eyelids flutter and want to close; four, the sun's warmth over your body is making your muscles loose and wide; five, you are there…

Your favourite trees are here. There's a beautiful blue pool with tiny rainbow-coloured fish darting here and there. Budding blossoms fill the air with fragrance and you recognize the fragrance as you breathe it in.

Your inner eye can see a peaceful garden, bringing into view all the things you love – the soft tickly grass, birds flying and swooping and singing. It's so natural. Listen to the noises of the garden; it soothes your brain automatically. Enjoy every part of your garden in your mind.

Allow yourself to enjoy it all. Think how wonderful and tranquil your garden is. You soak in the strength of the trees and the pleasure of being within a circle of trees, protected and cool. You fall asleep in the summer garden, feeling nourished and safe.

You are growing a tiny baby together … you are parents, emotionally and spiritually and physically nurturing a baby. Each parent has a great input into the spiritual well-being of a baby. Both of you wonder at the miracle of your baby's development. The baby feels these images and basks in them as you communicate emotions of love and safety. As a couple, you're looking forward to the day of the birth and knowing the early hours of your birthing day can be spent visualizing your garden in safe oblivion.

When you rest in your safe place during labour, this feeling of peace and calm that you create will balance your hormones and activate your parasympathetic nervous system, assisting in a rapid opening of your cervix. The balance between your sympathetic and parasympathetic nervous systems will ensure that your baby feels calm and happy, and as a result you, the mother, will feel calm and confident too. When the baby feels relaxed and balanced, the baby's brain secretes hormones of readiness and endorphins that command the mother's hypothalamus to excrete the birthing hormone, oxytocin. Moreover, the baby's placenta releases hormones that ensure that the cervix and the surrounding tissue are transformed into the consistency of softly-set jelly from 38 weeks onwards. So, by term, your pelvis will really feel like it is filled with softly-set jelly and that it is getting more and more jelly-like every day, reaching its maximum liquid jelly-like state during the actual delivery of the baby's head.

Visualize all of these changes while imagining that you are in your garden of relaxation. By enjoying and understanding the physical benefits of being very relaxed, you are allowing optimum quantities of helpful hormones to be released into your vaginal tissues, softening them on a daily basis, especially in the last few weeks of pregnancy.

It will be so easy for the top of your uterus to talk to your cervix because you have preprogrammed the pathways of communication. Special pathways, which run along the side walls of the uterus, will take the message to the cervix to become flatter and thinner and to dilate quickly. Your baby will assist the cervical dilatation by swiveling its little head into the cervix and pushing down lower and lower. As the top of your uterus contracts on the baby's bottom, it will help the cervix to open easily like an ever-expanding circle.

Keep flashing back to your garden in your mind, both between and during your contractions. Remember to take three deep breaths at the beginning of every contraction, as we have now made your three breaths an automatic conditioned response that relaxes all the muscles of your body. I also emphasize that it is equally important to take three deep breaths at every relaxation phase between contractions. This will ensure that your muscles relax twice as deeply, to release more endorphins and increase your sense of anesthesia. This in turn will help you to feel more comfort during your next contraction.

Imagine that you have just concluded a contraction…quickly click your eyelids closed and say 'I'm going into self-hypnosis and into total muscular relaxation', or 'I'm going to my special place, my garden of relaxation and into total muscular relaxation'. You are training your mind to go to this garden and relax immediately. Imagine again you are between contractions – open your eyes wide and fix your gaze on an imaginary spot then click them shut again when you are ready.

Every time you access your garden or other chosen safe place, this will bring a sense of peace to your nervous system and this calms the seat of your emotions within your brain – your hypothalamus. See the hypothalamus as a shimmering layer, like the surface of a blue lagoon, or a sheet of water across the middle of your brain at the level of your eyes. Imagine this shimmering layer of colour, so soothing and calming. A cool, calm hypothalamus will send cooling and calming influences to the whole of your body, helping your uterus to work in a calm and efficient manner.

Safe Place: Alternative Scenario (The Lift)

Because pain is not static during birth, but peaks and dips throughout the labour, I have found a lot of my mothers relate to safe places that involve movement. This one is a favourite:

- *As you feel your contraction come on: Imagine you are on the top floor of a very tall, old building. You walk over to the lift that seems to beckon you to walk in and you step in and close the old fashioned grille-like metal gates and press the button to go all the way down to the basement, which is ten levels below. As you descend down each level, your body gets heavier and heavier and you feel yourself relaxing more and more, reaching a deeper and deeper feeling of relaxation. By the time you reach the basement, ten levels below, your body is incredibly heavy and relaxed; as you leave the bustle of the outside world far, far behind, you feel very detached from the outside world. You have reached the basement of relaxation and you can enjoy it for as long as you like.*

- *As the contraction passes: Press the button for the lift to go back up to the top floor. On the very top floor, which has a glass roof, there is a beautiful glowing sunrise and you are drawn towards to it, feeling ever lighter and clearer with every floor you go up. You feel so light you could float, as though you're made of air.*

- *Continue going up and down the different comfort levels as and when you need to. Catch the fresh air as you go up and sink into sedation as you drop down to your basement of relaxation.*

Case History: Using a 'safe place' – Anne

I had been nervous about whether or not I would be able to retreat to my safe place during labour, but when contractions started three days after my due date, I was amazed at how easily I was able to slip into my safe place. Whenever a contraction came on, I automatically found myself visualizing jumping into a rock pool in the Scottish Highlands, which I had visited as a child and all but

---

forgotten about. It was the coldest water I'd ever been in, and as every contraction peaked, I imagined the freezing water numbing my body and taking the edge off them.

The biggest surprise to me was that I hadn't prepared the rock pools as my safe place, but a series of gardens with steps leading down to the sea. I guess that image was too passive for me and my mind needed a stronger 'anaesthetic' on the day, but it worked fantastically well for me and really made me aware of how powerfully the mind can control what the body feels.

Partner's Tip: The safe place as anaesthetic – the pinch test
To test the efficacy of the mother's safe place, let her become deeply relaxed. Stroke her arms and face gently downwards and talk her through her safe place visualization, inducing deeper and deeper relaxation. After a few minutes, take one of her arms and pinch the skin on the back of her hand, reasonably firmly. Gently replace her arm and continue to stroke her, before asking her to come back to full awareness. Then pinch the mother's hand with the same pressure as before. If she was properly relaxed, the pinch should feel significantly harder the second time. If it feels the same to her, then she needs to become more deeply relaxed and needs more practice. It may take time but everyone can do this in the end.

Preparing for Labour – Visualization
Bring your body into a state of deep muscle relaxation and go into self-hypnosis so that your mind is receptive to positive thoughts. You are now ready to move through a visualization. Through these mindscapes, you will condition your body to anticipate the demands and stages of pregnancy and labour, so that on the day it is familiar and as you have imagined, giving you confidence and emotional control, and reinforcing your belief in your ability to give birth. During the visualization, I encourage you and your partner to consider your body in a different way, journeying around it from the inside in order to demystify its role in the birthing process – this also encourages empathy with

your baby and is a powerful bonding tool. As foetal positioning is a crucial factor in the ease of a birth, we will visualize the baby adopting the correct position for birth within the womb – the occipito-anterior position in which the back of the baby's head (the occiput) is touching the pubic bones and the baby is facing your sacrum or backbone. You are encouraged to perceive the pelvic bones as soft, flexible, mobile structures that flare outwards easily to accommodate your baby's head as it engages.

This is a very bonding part of the programme and can be as creative as it is spiritual – I find many of my mothers really enjoy visualizing the birthing space in the pelvis being filled with soft jelly and of thinking of the pelvic muscles and ligaments as having the consistency of liquid. By considering the body in this naïve way, it's much easier to respond to mantras like 'your body is opening', 'your cervix is soft and slippery' – repetition is very effective here – and the results can be spectacular during labour.

Again, you may choose to record this transcript onto a tape cassette, or have it read to you (regularly) by the father or your birth partner. Remember that hypnotic speech is much softer and slower than normal speech patterns.

Pre-programming for Labour Script
Let your eyes fix on an imaginary point on the ceiling so that your eyelids are looking up. Be aware of your breathing. After a while your eyes will become heavy and drowsy and when you feel that you cannot keep your eyes open any longer, just let them close and take 3 deep breaths into the lowest part of your tummy. Say to yourself 'I am going into self-hypnosis now. I am going to my safe place' and as you do so, visualize your safe place and relax into your body. Each breath is travelling through your body – travelling to all the muscles in your body.

Work your way through your body, tightening and then fully relaxing every part of your body – your feet, calves, thighs... Now your bottom and your pelvic floor. As you relax your abdominal region I want you to honour these wonderful muscles that are cradling your baby. Imagine hugging your baby from the inside out, then let it go. With every breath, you are seeing these muscles relax more and more. The baby senses the wonderful space around it and it can flex its muscles, flex its limbs, taking advantage of the extra space that you provide by relaxing, dropping down into your pelvic space, its little head nestling there. Now I want you to imagine a golden light coming in through the top of your head, down through your body, relaxing and caressing your body as it moves. As your body fills with golden light, it is passed on through the placenta to your baby and your baby floats in the golden energy of love and peace. You feel deeply relaxed and serene.

When you awaken on the day that your baby is going to be born, you will remember this deep, intimate sensation and it will make you feel calm and relaxed, as though this was just like any other day of your life. You will be pleased and surprised that you feel so calm and in control of your emotions, and you will know that you can feel calm and relaxed – just as you do now – all the way through your birth process. The neck of your womb will release a lovely discharge, pink in colour, which is a lubricating agent for your baby to slip through, and the whole of your vagina will be slippery and soft and moist, making it easy for your baby's head to slip out of your body.

You will feel the contractions come and go at 10-minute intervals, and will be surprised to note that they feel very much like the Braxton-Hicks contractions that you are feeling now in these last months of your pregnancy. You note these practise contractions and let them float away, and the only difference you will feel during the birth is that the contractions will be regular and organized in such a way that you experience each one as a firm tightening that begins at the top of your uterus and travels downwards like a wave, pushing your baby down towards the lowest part of your vaginal opening.

The top of your uterus is an interesting and automatic muscle that contracts and relaxes, like a rubbery dome which is pushed down and then springs back immediately into a relaxed state. During the birth, you will be able to use into deep hypnosis to allow fresh supplies of blood, oxygen and sugar to reach every part of the uterine muscle, even the tiniest part of the uterine muscle, so that it is comfortable. Remember the more oxygen that your uterus gets, the more comfortable your uterine contractions will feel to you. So as you breathe deeply and generously, both during and between all your contractions, your uterus will feel more and more comfortable as you progress.

As the top of your uterus contracts, you will also feel a warm sensation of expansion around your hip and pelvic areas, like a ripple flowing outwards with absolutely no aim any more. You will feel a sensation of openness and your pelvis will feel warm and loose. You will know that your pelvis is widening and the opening in your body is getting wider with every contraction. Remember that as the top of your uterus squeezes on your baby's bottom, this pressure will be transmitted vertically to your baby's head. Your baby's head will automatically press down into the inner aspect of your cervix, encouraging it to become thinner and thinner and more and more open. You know that the purpose of the contractions is to push your baby out of your body and you know that your body is designed for, and capable of, giving birth.

You also know – and can see – that as the top of your uterus contracts, special messages flow down from the top of the uterus to the side walls of your cervix. With every contraction, there is a very definite relaxation and further opening of the cervix. The gentlest of contractions will programme your cervix to immediately respond by dilating easily. And even between the contractions, your cervix will keep on dilating, so that within a very short time, it will be fully dilated, making your labour shorter and more comfortable.

As your labour progresses, your baby's head will drop easily, as the tissues in your pelvis and vagina change into the consistency of softly-set jelly. Once you pass 38 weeks, your cervix will become thinner, flatter and more stretchable. You will also have asked your baby's head to form into a slightly oblong shape to mould down confidently into the pelvis and snuggle into your cervix. As your baby's head pushes into your cervix, it will make the cervix even thinner and this will help the cervix to become dilated in a very short time.

You will confidently push your baby out of your body because you know that there is a lot of space around your baby's head. The skin of your perineum will become more and more elastic, and you will sense the lower part of your body becoming very soft and warm, silky and elastic. In a short time you will feel your baby dropping down low within your vagina, its spine running down the length of your tummy, so that you will feel an urge to push your baby out of your body. If you imagine a wide channel between your thighs, you will feel your vagina slowly dilate, bit by bit, in a calm manner that allows your baby to be born gently.

You will feel so in control of your thoughts and emotions that you will be able to confidently and fully participate in the experience of your body gently opening to release your baby into the world. You will know there is a very small gap between your baby's head and the outside world, and a few gentle, efficient contractions are all that will be needed for your baby to be born.

After a short while, you will feel a lovely fullness in the lower part of your body. The gentle pressure on your back passage will indicate to you that the baby is going to be born, and it will make you very excited. It will make you smile and look at your partner with confidence and excitement as you share the magic moment just before the final contraction that brings your baby into your arms and makes you parents. As you receive and hold your baby in your arms, you and your partner will hold your baby gently to your breast, to your skin, touching and kissing and looking at your baby and speaking to your baby, welcoming your baby so happily into this world. And this loving welcome will be imprinted into your baby for life.

The umbilical cord will not be cut until the cord stops pulsating and as your baby nuzzles into the skin of your breast, the uterus will contract very firmly, expelling the placenta to the outside with very little blood loss. Your uterus will remain safely contracted from then on, regaining its former natural shape within a few days. Breastfeeding will be established immediately, with instant let down of colostrum, your nourishing first breast milk. You and your partner will form a very close-knit bond with your baby and you'll be bonded in love forever.

You have just walked through your baby's birth. Every part of you tingles with joy and anticipation that everything you have visualized will be your reality. You feel safe now that you have done the preparation and know what to expect of the labour process, and you know everything you ask of your body will happen. Moreover, when both mother and father believe and practise this approach, it works twice as well, and your baby grows within this belief system and feels safe. Take a deep breath in and out, and slowly come to full awareness in your own time.

Visualization tip: Thinning cervix

From week 38, begin short daily visualization exercises that concentrate on your cervix opening and thinning. The thinner it is when you go into labour, the more easily it will dilate to 10cm when the baby's head starts to bear down. This reduces pain, and also cuts down the amount of time spent in labour.

Birth Story: Lapse in mental concentration leading to interrupted labour – Uma

It was 3 weeks before my due date and I attended one of Gowri's self-hypnosis classes. I had just gone on maternity leave and was looking forward to the next three weeks rest. I didn't feel relaxed at all as I had just been through a stressful period of conflict with my mother-in-law. On the journey home from the class, I felt quite strange and the first contractions started as soon as I stepped into the house. I pottered about, packing the recycling bags and breathing low into my belly – just as we had been doing in the class. In truth, I felt as if I was still in the trance state that I had been in during the class, because as the contractions grew stronger, I simply felt more relaxed. Everything was perfectly fine and for a couple more hours I was easily slipping into a quiet trance state with every contraction.

At about 1am, my husband called the midwives, just to let them know things had been ticking along nicely since 9pm, but that I was still relaxed enough to chat.

They soon came round and by 2.30am, it seemed as if the baby was ready to be born. But just then, my elder son awoke with teething pain and cried out for me. On reflection, I think we should simply have brought him down to us, but instead we sent up his uncle to soothe him. In the end, my husband went up to him and stayed with him for about 2 hours.

Downstairs, the labour process seemed to slow right down and although the contractions continued, by 4am, there was still no sign of the baby. It was clear my concern for my son was hindering my labour.

By the time my husband came back downstairs, I was feeling tired, but I continued to use the self-hypnosis techniques throughout, and rested well between the contractions – it was a magical time of quiet and gentle focus.

By 8am, the labour had slowed down so much the midwives thought it best if they left, and my brother took my son out for a walk to the park. The sound of the front door closing, together with the sight of the midwives ready to leave seemed to re-start the labour immediately.

I stood up to say goodbye to the midwives, when my waters broke explosively and water gushed out. From that point onwards there were only a few contractions as the baby moved down and out. The birthing stage was rapid. The baby's head was born after only a couple of big contractions and then his body followed ten seconds later. He weighed 8lb 4oz and was in fine health. No tears, or grazes. I felt completely comfortable afterwards and found the birthing experience really empowering.

Emotional Preparation

Bonding with your Baby

'The exact moment of the beginning of personhood, is at the exact moment of conception'

DR MCCARTHY DE MERE

MD AND LAW PROFESSOR AT TENNESSEE UNIVERSITY

Bonding with your baby isn't something that begins at birth. From the moment you learn you're pregnant, bonding can begin. Even when your baby is an embryo, not yet a foetus or recognizable baby, we believe there's a soul there. And that means someone to love.

From day one, when a pregnant woman registers with me, I call her a mother, and her partner, a father. By encouraging her to consider herself a mother even before the baby is born, the mother learns to accept her new role and extends a welcome to the baby. Her role as nurturer, life-giver and provider has already begun and it is during her pregnancy that she is given the opportunity to cherish this in an emotional capacity. Once the baby is born, the parent's role becomes much more physical – the acts of feeding, changing nappies, cradling to sleep and so on. It is a tiring and hectic time, but without exception, it is always so much more joyous when the emotional groundwork is already in place.

There are so many ways to love your baby in the womb. Consider some of these little intimacies for introducing yourselves to each other:

- Humanize your baby – don't call him/her 'it'. Choose a nickname that is loving, fond and intimate. It doesn't need to reflect your real name choices, or even be unisex. Some mothers are concerned that they'll get so used to a pregnancy nickname that it will stick, but this is rarely the case. Once there's a little face looking up at you, your baby takes on a different character and will rapidly inhabit his or her proper name.
- Lather and hug your bump in the shower.
- Stroke your baby bump at every opportunity – it's especially great when the midwives record the baby's position and you know where to place your hand to feel for the baby's face, bottom, hands or feet. You may even get a little kick or prod as a reward.
- Try gently humming your favourite lullaby or tune. The soft reverberations massage and relax the baby and, chances are, it will be instantly soothing to your baby when out of the womb.
- Send love hormones to your baby. There is a constant interchange of endorphins between the two of you and the more you can communicate warmth, love and safety to your baby, the more they will send back to you. Consider yourself a little team looking out for each other.
- Pore over the scan photos. It's uncanny how much newborn babies look like their 20-week-plus scan photos. The shape of their head, profile, lips, nose, will all correspond to the tender little newborn in your arms.
- Try to have a new thought about your baby every day. Imagine your first walk together, or your first bath, the joy of breastfeeding, or the delight of that first smile. Every milestone you anticipate with your baby will fill you with delight, and your baby too.
- When deeply relaxed, visualize your baby floating in your tummy, bathed in a glorious white light. You might like to imagine the colour changing to blue to pink to yellow, or perhaps just brightening in intensity. Feel still, pure and light as your baby's new life flourishes inside you.

The following poem, by a famous Indian poet, was given to me by one of my mothers and encapsulates the magical bond between parent and child. A great many of my mothers have since been enchanted by its purity and have found that its sentiments echo and articulate their own feelings, reinforcing the bonding process.

'Where have I come from, where did you discover me?'
the baby asked its mother.
She answered, half crying, half laughing, and clasping the baby to her breast:
'You were hidden in my heart as its desire, my darling;
You were in the dolls of my childhood games.
And when with clay I made the image of my God every morning,
I made and unmade you.
Then you were enshrined with our household deity.
In his worship, I worshipped you.
In all my hopes and my loves, in life
In the life of my mother you have lived.
In the lap of the deathless spirit who rules our home
You have been nursed for ages.
When in my girlhood my heart was opening its petals
You hovered as a fragrance about it.
Your tender softness bloomed in my youthful limbs
Like a glow in the sky before sunrise.
Heaven's first darling, twin born with the afternoon light
You have floated down the stream of the world's life
And at last you have stranded on my heart;
As I gaze on your face, mystery overwhelms me:
You, who belong to all, have become mine.
For fear of losing you, I hold you tight to my breast.
What magic has snared the world's treasure in these slender arms of mine?

RABINDRANATH TAGORE

Birth story: The sceptic – Carol

I never would have thought that after the induction/pethidine/epidural/forceps delivery of my first baby two years ago, I would enjoy giving birth to my second child. But I did.

After the technological nightmare of my first delivery, I became interested in a water birth, so the hospital put me in touch with Dr Motha. I went for a consultation expecting to find a doctor behind a desk with a list of technical specifications on temperature maintenance and sub-aqua monitoring. To my dismay, I was seated on a cushion and told I was to be given a lesson in 'self-hypnosis,' which didn't appeal to me at all. However, I soon discovered that this bore no relation to my somewhat sinister idea of hypnotism, but is a way of teaching conscious relaxation.

In the classes, Dr Motha told us that the uterus is a strong muscle specifically designed for the labour process – let it work without tension, let the muscles relax and you can allow the baby to slip through easily and comfortably. We learnt to relax our bodies completely and at will, and learnt to think positively and joyfully about the birth of our babies. This was fine in theory – and admittedly the relaxing cured my bad back – but would it help me get through labour? I still didn't really believe it. When my waters broke at 4pm one afternoon, I went to hospital, even though I didn't have any contractions. I was strapped up to a monitoring device but by 11pm nothing was happening, so the doctors decided to admit me to the antenatal ward with a view to inducing me the next morning – exactly what I'd been fearing all along.

On my own in the ward, I decided to stop fretting and do something positive. I sat in a dark corner and relaxed as we'd been taught, shutting off everything around me and concentrating on letting myself open up, welcoming my baby. By midnight I was being hustled back down the stairs by a nurse who refused to wait for the lift; 'Hold on dear, we don't want you having it up here.' I'd gone to

6cm dilatation in less than an hour, and it was only when I realized that I should call a midwife and start trying to cope with the hospital scene again that it began to hurt.

Once left on my own in a delivery room, I stood leaning on the bed, which immediately helped – sitting or lying down was excruciating – and I started to calm down again. My husband and Dr Motha arrived together and I relaxed still further, knowing they would now deal with the outside world for me. Dr Motha turned down the lights and gave my husband directions on how to set up the pool. I was still a little frightened by the pain I'd felt and my body was trembling with the pressure of standing. The relief getting into the pool was immediate as the warm water took my weight and soothed me.

I soon found a rhythm, kneeling in the water, leaning my head on my arms on the side, breathing deeply as each contraction did its work. I concentrated on keeping my muscles, soft and loose and opening to help my baby. I could feel each contraction and was aware of the effort my body was making and the effect it was having, but felt no pain.

Between contractions, I enjoyed the water, a smile, a drink; when the urge to push came, Dr Motha reminded me just to breathe deeply. There was no need to set my teeth and strain. I could feel the baby's head coming down a little further each time, gently opening his way into the world. If I'd tried to force him, I would have torn.

At that moment, I did feel a sudden, sharp pain and thought I must be nearly there. I put my hand down to feel how much further I had to go, and felt the baby's head! The next contraction came, caught me unready, I yelled, the baby yelled, my husband yelled 'You've done it!', and I was standing up, to take my baby from Dr Motha, feeling exulted and incredulous that it could all be over so soon, so beautifully. My baby nuzzled me and smiled.

Later, my husband and Dr Motha left and the midwife went to fetch a wheelchair to take me to the post-natal ward. I could have taken the stairs two at a time, but she insisted that I sit down.

Perhaps she felt she had to do something other than check the heartbeat and write up the notes. That was when I heard the woman in the next room, shrieking and sobbing in the accepted, expected way of 'media' childbirth.

And I wanted to tell her – there is another way, a way so old that after centuries of innovation, research and drugs testing, we're having to rediscover it. Your baby knows what to do, your body knows what to do – there's nothing to fear but fear itself.

Generating Emotional Calm and Control

By studying the techniques of deep muscle relaxation, self-hypnosis and visualization, you have all the mental tools you need for your body to welcome the mechanics of labour, and for your mind to float away. By the time you go into labour – six, five, four, three months from now – you will have become adept at controlling your own levels of self-hypnosis and deep muscle relaxation. You know exactly what to expect, your body is primed and birthfit, and the birth carries no fear for you. Instead you feel excited, in control and capable.

So with all this in mind, I want you to tap into this positivity and really bask in the deep, beautiful emotions you harbour for your baby, because in the following visualization – a birth rehearsal – we are going to prepare to meet your baby. Up until now, you have been viewing the birth theoretically, as a logical physical function. Now, in your final months of pregnancy, I want you to begin to anticipate the emotions involved in actually meeting your baby – what it's going to be like to hold him or her in your arms and look into those deep limpid eyes. Consider how your love for your baby can help you during the birth; it is a very powerful tool. A positive mental attitude can help you greatly in how you interpret and deal with pain – for example, by regarding every contraction as a push that brings your baby closer to meeting you, you are far more likely to accept, and even welcome, the tightenings.

As your due date comes closer you should be listening to the Birth Rehearsal Script (see below) as often as you can (daily if possible) especially after week 36. If you made the cassette tape as suggested on page 94, you could add it to the end of side B and listen to all the transcripts together. However, you may like to make another tape for the latter stages of your pregnancy and labour. Together with the Birth Rehearsal Script you could add the Pre-programming for Labour Script (pages 112–16) and the Secret Garden or Lift Visualization Scripts (page 110). This tape is good to listen to as soon as your labour starts – it can powerfully encourage your body through contractions and help speed up dilation. For those readers who would like more direct help, the Jeyarani Labour tape is available (see Appendix C, page 313).

Birth Rehearsal Script

On the day of the birth you wake knowing that 'This will be the day I see my baby face to face'. Go within yourself and see the baby. Your brain and spinal cord will release huge amounts of endorphins because you have practised this and so the endorphins are released automatically.

The first droplets of birth hormones are released. There is a tightness in the top of your uterus sending a wave down to the cervix, widening it. You experience period-like sensations. On the first contraction, the top of the uterus contracts, which firmly nudges the baby's head down towards the lowest part of the cervix. The baby pushes the cervix, moulding into it and making it dilate easily like flattened dough, with a central hole about 2cm wide. These early contractions are 10–15 minutes apart but are so light you are hardly able to register them consciously. However, even the softest of contractions is programmed to gently open your cervix. Special message fibres from the pacemakers of your uterus flow down to the cervix to open it more and more. The spaces between the contractions are generous enough to allow you to drift off to your safe place in your mind. When the next contraction comes it feels so distant and natural – you're safe in the knowledge that even the most gentle contractions are still opening your cervix more and more. Contractions in the early stages only last about 30 seconds, so your inner mind feels safe enough to doze or even sleep through them.

With every one of your uterine waves, you are able to take your mind into self-hypnosis, into your safe place. Take three deep breaths at the beginning of each contraction and give the command 'open'. Speak to your partner and say, 'My contractions have started.' Your partner gently strokes your head or arms; he snuggles up to you, saying 'Relax'. You snuggle up through all the contractions.

The baby's head is being pushed into the middle of your pelvis. You confidently note that as the baby is comfortably moving down into the ever-widening circle of bones you remain in a gentle, deep trance state. Remember your body can mould: 70 per cent of your body is in fact water and 40 per cent of your pelvic bones are also made of water. The cervix is opening more and more. The baby's head is dropping down into the vaginal space. The vaginal muscles are dilating in a large circle, which is becoming purely elastic. As the cervix dilates, so does your vagina, your perineum and all the birthing places.

You and your baby are working as a team, and the baby sends more stimulus to your pituitary gland, which then releases more oxytocin. You notice only that the contractions are regular, comfortable and relaxing. Every breath you take releases endorphins – comfortably anaesthetizing your body, and every breath also releases softening hormones from the baby's placenta, making your pelvis soft and generous.

The contractions are now 5 minutes apart and you notice that you feel very comfortable. You are deeply entranced by the relaxation created by yourself and your partner. You are feeling safe and secure. You handled the early contractions so well that, due to your conditioning, your inner mind now tells your brain that you can handle stronger contractions – twice as much as before and the baby is pushed further into your birthing space.

When the contractions come at 5-minute intervals, and are stronger, it is probably time to go to your birthing unit or, if you are giving birth at home, to call the midwife. You relax while the bags are packed in the car and you remain in a trance, eyes half closed as you are guided to the car and settle in the seat. Your partner drives you to the hospital and you feel relaxed and confident. Everything you see along the way, street lights, traffic signals, shop signs all take you even deeper into muscle relaxation and release more endorphins. On arrival at the birthing unit, the midwife is very pleased to see mother and father so relaxed. She examines you and tells you how wonderfully strong your baby's heartbeat is and this relaxes you even more. She also tells you that your cervix is so thin and well-dilated that it is amazing. The baby's head has already dropped down.

You continue to relax more and more and, when you are ready, you might like to slip into a birthing pool or take a shower or a short bath. The contact of the water has a wonderful effect on the buttocks and back, which automatically relax as the blood supply improves dramatically. Moreover, the warmth of the water increases the blood flow into your cervix and the cervix dilates easily and willingly. Your cervix is also responsive to hormones from the placenta and it becomes even looser and wider and the baby's head drops down further.

You are beginning to feel that the baby is pushing onto your back passage and you notice an urge to empty your bowels and as you communicate that feeling, your midwife smiles and examines you and says that you are now ready to push. You feel a great sense of excitement and pride and you know you will now see your baby very soon.

You get into the birthing position – on your side, or squatting, or on all fours, or in a supported squat. If you are having your baby in water, all you have to do is continue squatting and pushing in a downwards movement. Your strong uterus pushes firmly down, down to a jelly-like and elastic vagina where your baby's head is going to emerge. Your vaginal muscles relax in ever-widening circles and the vaginal opening relaxes easily to allow your baby to come out quickly and easily.

At the peak of every contraction you take a long deep breath and push down. Between contractions, you are able to relax, lie back and breathe in deeply. When the contraction comes, you get into your pushing position again. These waves are twice as powerful, but you perceive them as being twice as comfortable. As you have each contraction, there is a strong impulse to push and you are rewarded by feeling the baby's head easing its way down your jelly-like vaginal muscles. The support you have from your partner and midwife gives you deep trust and you feel very relaxed, so more and more of your baby's head comes down. Everyone around you encourages you and then, with another contraction, you push really hard and a rush of adrenalin flows through you – you've done it!

You reach down and touch your baby's head. With the next contraction your baby's shoulders, body, legs and feet emerge too. Your loving arms reach out and you're bringing your baby up to your heart. As soon as the baby's body is exposed to the cool air, it takes a quick and confident breath. Within three to four deep breaths, the baby is a breathing individual in its own right.

You and your partner look at the baby's face. You wonder at the beauty of your baby and your little baby laps up the praise, love and delight that you both show. You express your delight as you thank your baby for being your baby. Your baby's mind is deeply imprinted with your loving welcome. You are all transported in a bubble of happiness, which will last forever. Your love radiates out to join the other happy mothers and fathers everywhere.

The baby is still attached to you by the umbilical cord, and so you and your baby share oxygen and endorphins. When the cord stops pulsating, it is easily clamped and cut by the father. After delivery, your uterus firmly contracts and the entire placenta peels from the inner wall of your uterus and slips away into your vagina. You push once more and the soft placenta slides out and the midwife tells you all the parts of the placenta are complete

and intact. The midwife examines you and says that you have an intact per-
ineum and vagina, and you feel a great sense of pride and relief. You feel that
your body has done exactly what your mind wanted it to do. You did it. When
you are ready, your baby suckles at your breast instinctively and everyone
exclaims how wonderfully well you've done.

Case History: Using gentle 'intervention' – Maria

Maria was overdue and the hospital had induced her by breaking her waters. She was in labour all day, at only 1cm dilatation, until eventually she called me saying the midwives wanted to put her on a drip to speed up the contractions. I went to the hospital and tried to get her put in a pool, but none were available, not even a bath. So I took her to the shower and sprayed warm water over her tummy, and up and down her back, focusing particularly on the sacrum. All the while I was softly repeating 'your cervix is opening, the baby is moving down', like a mantra – over and over and over.

After about an hour and a half of this, she asked to come out of the shower because she felt an overwhelming urge to push. I couldn't believe it could be the baby already, but called the mid-wife anyway – who promptly threw Maria's husband, Andrew, and me out of the room while she did the examination. It was very quiet and Andrew was nervously pacing up and down the corridor until he couldn't stand it any more and went to check on his wife's progress. Maria was fully dilated and already pushing! Three push-es later they had a baby girl. In this instance, the combination of the standing position, warm water and the visualization of her cervix opening led Maria to dilate 9cm in 90 minutes.

Labour visualization tip
Think of every contraction as a wave that washes your baby further down the birth passages. Welcome each one for bringing your baby closer to you.

Father's tip: Visualizations to hasten labour
Choose a helpful phrase such as 'every breath you take is making you more and more relaxed' and repeat it like a mantra in a low, soft voice, while your partner is in self-hypnosis. Focus on encouraging her body to open up by making positive suggestions such as 'your cervix is opening', 'your hips are getting wider and looser', 'your birthing space is getting softer and silkier', 'your cervix is thin and slippery and is sliding open magically'.

Be creative – choose soft, sensuous words that are easily accepted by her mind and body. Don't worry if it feels repetitive or you think it sounds boring to her, she will let you know if it annoys her. Subtle, positive, loving suggestions made to the receptive mind can have a really dramatic effect on the body.

SECTION B

The month-by-month programme

Introduction to the Programme

So this is it – the first step on the road to meeting your baby. Everything you read on the following pages is intended to gear your body towards birthfitness and, in so doing, create a calm, clear sanctuary for your baby. It's an enormously bonding process – you'll find that your baby kicks with delight during the pelvic drainage massage in the Creative Healing treatments, for example, because babies love the boost of freshly oxygenated blood they receive.

And although the treatments have very real – and quantifiable – health benefits, they are also crucial opportunities for you to feel physically cosseted and emotionally cherished. They allow you to step out of the routine and bustle of your everyday life and dwell purely on your blooming baby; so enjoy these quiet times while you can – this is one of your last chances for me-time before (and after!) your baby comes along.

Most of my mothers embark on the treatment programme at about 16 weeks. This is because many mothers don't discover they're pregnant until they're about 6–8 weeks, and it often takes a little while for the news to sink in and for them to become pro-active about it. Also, side effects such as vomiting and tiredness tend to have settled down by week 16, which is an important consideration with regards to the diet – a heightened sense of smell and nausea can make it difficult to follow a balanced diet in the early weeks, so it is unrealistic to expect mothers to exclude wheat and sugar in addition to foods that make them queasy. However, I have found that by weeks 12–16, mothers feel mentally and physically ready to begin getting birthfit.

Of course, I'm delighted when mothers enrol on the programme before 16 weeks, as it can only ever be beneficial to them. However, until the placenta becomes firmly attached to the uterus (by week 12) there are certain treatments that should be avoided, but I detail these clearly in each month's section and there are so many other, gentle methods you can follow until that time which can help abate all the unpleasant side-effects. (If you discover you are pregnant very early on and wish to begin a treatment, I advise Reiki, as it is the least intrusive form of healing.)

To allow for those of you who can't wait to get started, I have devised the programme to start on month two, working on the assumption that you discover you are pregnant after your first missed period, at about 5–6 weeks. If you prefer to start a few weeks later, simply pick up the programme at your corresponding week of gestation. You don't need to worry about 'making up' the previous sessions.

When can you really say that you became pregnant?
Most clinicians count the beginning of your pregnancy from the first day of your last menstrual period. But in reality your baby is just implanting and is a little ball of cells at week 4 in your cycle and is really only 2 weeks on from fertilization and coming into being. Even so, your baby is still there. Dr Hymie Gordon, Chairman of the Department of Genetics at the Mayo Clinic points out that 'By all the criteria of modern molecular biology, life is present from the moment of conception'.

There Are No Shortcuts

The programme is comprehensive from the outset, and some mothers find this a bit of a shock. Often this is because the news of their pregnancy has made them less active – sometimes prompted by fears of miscarriage – and more self-indulgent with their diet, so the contrast is heightened. But even if you're raring to go, there is still a steep curve when embarking on the programme. From a standing start, I ask you to start doing gentle daily exercise, restrict your diet, take herbal supplements, and book in for physical treatments. There are certain elements of the programme – like the treatments – that are modular and incorporated only at specific points in the pregnancy, but most of the preparation begins here and carries on until you deliver.

There is a good reason for there being no shortcuts in this programme. If you start an intensive exercise programme, you would not expect to see a difference to your figure for several weeks. Similarly, the Gentle Birth Method trains your body for something even more radical – a physiological and physical change. We're not only aiming for your uterus to be detoxified, we want it to be as toned as any of your leg, shoulder, arm or stomach muscles; we want the muscles in your pelvis to become so soft that the inner diameter of the pelvic cavity becomes measurably wider; we want your cervix not only to be decongested, but also thin. And this doesn't take weeks – it takes months.

The difficulty for you is that you can't see the changes. Stomach crunches may give you a noticeably flat tummy at the gym, but of course, you can't see how well the Ayurvedic herbs are toning your uterus. So you've got to take a leap of faith. Your motivation and reward is a short, gentle birth and it can be yours if you build up your birthfitness steadily. Look at the figures below – they clearly prove that the more you do to train your body now, the more your body will be able to respond positively during labour:

How Gentle Birth Method figures compare to national averages

Vaginal Birth rate:

National average	Gentle Birth Method	
77.6%	>4 treatments: 85.2%	>9 treatments: 90.6%

Caesarean Section rate:

National average	Gentle Birth Method	
22.4%	>4 treatments: 14.7%	>9 treatments: 9.4%

Epidural rate:

National average	Gentle Birth Method	
33%	>4 treatments: 30.5%	>9 treatments: 17.2%

Instrumentation rate:

National average	Gentle Birth Method	
11%	4–8 treatments: 6.9%	>9 treatments: 6.1%

Episiotomy rate:

National average	Gentle Birth Method	
15%	4–8 treatments: 7.8%	>9 treatments: 3.4%

Intact Perineum rate:

National average	Gentle Birth Method	
Not Known	4–8 treatments: 67.2%	>9 treatments: 96.6%

Getting Started

- At the back of this book, and on www.gentlebirthmethod.com, you will find a list of practitioners who are trained in the Gentle Birth Method and know the programme. If possible, make an appointment with them for an initial consultation, where they will take your medical history (e.g. history of back pain or high blood pressure) and discuss with you the different elements of the programme.
- If there isn't a local Jeyarani practitioner in your area, don't worry. Find a local therapist you feel comfortable with, and are happy to see on a regular basis over the course of your pregnancy. They may not offer all the treatments advised in the programme, but in order of importance you want to find someone who can perform Reflexology, and ideally Creative Healing.

It is important that the therapist is happy to follow the programme with you, working from this book and not free-styling. Regardless of how experienced they may be in their field, the programme is not simply about having holistic treatments throughout your pregnancy. A back massage may be relaxing, but it will not necessarily get you birthfit.

This programme has been developed over 16 years and each treatment has a different physiological 'intention' at each stage of the pregnancy – so, for instance, when you have Creative Healing on a fortnightly basis, the therapist will be focusing on a different area, or emphasizing a different technique each time.

- If your therapist is happy to proceed, please ask them to contact the Jeyarani Centre (see Appendix C) for a therapist's information pack. Even if they do not already offer Creative Healing, we can supply short training courses and a teaching DVD so that they can learn the basic skills should they wish.
- Take this book to every appointment with your therapist, so that you are both working from the same programme.
- Make advance block-bookings, if you have to, to ensure you get appointments at the intervals detailed in the monthly timetable.
- Always speak to your therapist about any pains or problems you are experiencing, before commencing a treatment session.
- Remember that your partner or a friend can be the 'practitioner' and can administer some of the treatments on you. See Home Massage Treatments, Section A, pages 53–71. The Creative Healing DVD is also available (see Appendix C, page 314).

Note: I have suggested treatments for each week of your pregnancy. However, this may not be easy to implement. If as a rough guide you receive one-on-one treatments every fortnight throughout your pregnancy you will be well prepared. And remember, treatments alone cannot override the ill effects of a bad eating plan, so beware.

First Trimester

Month 2 (weeks 5–8)

Physical Preparation: Diet
Throughout this month:
- Limit yourself to a small glass (150ml) of pure fruit juice and three fruits (no bananas, grapes or mango) per day.
- Cut out sugar and refined carbohydrates, for example, cakes, biscuits, chocolate, puddings. If you crave something sweet, you can have two tea-spoons of honey per day as a spread on rice or oatcakes. Do not add honey into drinks that are too hot as this changes the nature of the honey and makes it toxic.
- Exclude wheat from your diet – look for alternatives such as rye bread, corn pasta, potato, barley or oats.

Note: As a compromise in the early months, you can have some sugar or wheat just one day a week. But please be careful and support the good work you've achieved in the previous six days.

- Limit carbohydrates to one portion per meal – one small cup of cooked carbohydrates such as rice, corn or quinoa.

- For every portion of carbohydrates, balance it with three portions of vegetables as recommended for your body type (see Ayurvedic section, pages 20–28).
- Ginger infusion: If you are beginning to feel tired and nauseous you may find it helpful to sip moderately warm Ginger Tea (see page 300). You can have this very supportive drink throughout your pregnancy, as it is a great balancer for all body types.
- Drink 2 litres (3½ pints) water daily. This should be at room temperature, as iced water or iced drinks shock the stomach, the pancreas and the vagus nerve that supplies the gut. (The pancreas is directly behind your stomach.) This cold shock causes poor secretions of the pancreatic enzymes leading to indigestion, food fermentation and resultant bloating in your gut.
- Avoid fizzy and commercial drinks – they are too high in sugar and artificial sweeteners. Fizzy drinks are carbonated. Carbonic acid depletes calcium from your gut and system, and can remove calcium from your bones. During pregnancy you need all the calcium that you can get.
- Limit your caffeine intake – caffeine encourages water retention and is associated with a higher risk of miscarriage in the first trimester.
- Remember, you only need 200 extra calories per day during pregnancy.
- Supplements: If you are not already on vitamins start taking prenatal vitamins, minerals and trace elements, as these are important for the development of the baby's organs (organo-genesis). Please check Appendix C for recommended brands.
- If possible, follow the Homoeopathic Tissue Salt Programme (see page 12). For the second month this is Calc. Fluor. 6c, Mag. Phos. 6c and Ferr. Phos 6c. Take one of each twice a day all through the month. If you live near a homoeopathic pharmacy they will be able to combine the tissue salts into one tablet for you. Alternatively, these are available from the Jeyarani clinic.
- Avoid alcohol and smoking cigarettes.

Physical Preparation: Exercise
Throughout this month:
- Do light exercise for 20 minutes per day. This could be a brisk walk from the shops, getting off the bus a stop earlier, or going for a light swim.

Note: recently there have been concerns about the effects of chlorinated water on pregnant women, as well as suggested links to asthma. Therefore I recommend swimming no more than once a week in a chlorinated pool; try to find an ozone-treated pool to swim in instead.

- Avoid yoga – it is generally not recommended in the first 3 months but can be gently introduced between 14 and 16 weeks of pregnancy.
- Avoid intense physical activity such as jogging or other strenuous sports.

Mental Preparation: Self-hypnosis

- If you can, do an introductory self-hypnosis course of four classes (see Appendix C). Even at this early stage in your pregnancy self-hypnosis and visualization helps to you to bond with your baby and makes you realize that there is a purpose to all the symptoms that you may be experiencing.
- Record onto audio tape the transcripts for the self-hypnosis and visualization techniques, detailed in Section A, pages 95–116. Start listening to the tape as often as possible. This will help you practise being able to switch off and go into self-hypnosis and establish your confidence early in your ability to give birth.
- Your baby's central nervous system is developing in your internal environment of peace, love and joy. Your baby feels all your feelings. You wish to only give your baby pleasant stimuli from the very beginning of pregnancy. You imprint your baby's nervous system from conception, so try to avoid arguments and stressful situations.

Week-by-week Progress and Treatment Recommendations

Week 5

Your baby has implanted and is still called an embryo at this stage. Your baby is only the size of a raisin. By day 21 the baby's heart has started to beat, the placenta begins to function and your baby's brain begins to develop. The spinal cord also grows rapidly giving your baby the appearance of having a little tail.

Recommended Treatment   Reiki (60 min.)

Week 6

Your embryo is just 5mm long and the beginnings of a little heart tube have already formed. There is detectable heartbeat on an ultrasound scan.

Recommended Treatment   Creative Healing (60 min.)

Note for Practitioner Week 6

Creative Healing: General treatment applied to the neck and back (see page 55–64); abdominal toning to reduce stretching pains associated with growing uterus and stretching of the round ligament (see pages 66–9); liver treatment; pancreatic treatment to ensure optimum digestion during crucial organo-genesis phase. Also possibly neck treatment to prevent/treat headaches common in early pregnancy and hiatus hernia treatment if mother shows signs of reflux.

Week 7

Your baby is continuing to develop and their facial features can be identified, including the mouth and tongue. The skeletal muscles are beginning to form and your baby begins to move. The blood circulatory system is forming and the heart is beginning to take shape. Your baby even has a blood type.

Recommended Treatments   Creative Healing (45 min.)

                                          + Reiki or Reflexology (45 min.)

In addition to Creative Healing, Reiki is wonderful as a general supportive measure if you have no symptoms; if you have severe nausea and vomiting, have a reflexology treatment.

Note for Practitioner Week 7

Creative Healing: General treatment (pages 55–64), back and spine treatments (pages 64–6) the heart and hiatus hernia treatments for the same indications as week 6.

Reflexology: This can be given if there is severe nausea and vomiting. Care must be taken to avoid working on the reflexes in the feet that represent the uterine area. The uterine area is situated on the inner aspect of the foot between the ankle and heel. However, massaging the ovarian area on the outer aspect of the ankle will help to balance the ovarian hormones that are produced from the Corpus Luteum of the ovary from ovulation to 16 weeks of pregnancy.

Week 8

Your baby is over a centimetre (½ in) long! The baby is floating around in a well-defined amniotic sac and looks like a little baby already, swimming and jumping movements are noted.

Recommended Treatment   None – Rest Week

Important note: Treatments to be careful about early on in pregnancy Reflexology treatments: it is imperative your therapist keeps away from the uterine areas on the foot, until the placenta is firmly implanted at 16 weeks.

Month 3 (weeks 9–12)

Physical Preparation: Diet
Throughout this month:

- Exclude wheat from your diet – look for alternatives such as rice, corn, quinoa, millet-based breakfast cereals, rye bread, corn pasta, barley or oats.
- Limit carbohydrates to one portion per meal – one cup of cooked rice or the equivalent.
- For every portion of carbohydrates, balance it with three portions of vegetables.

- Limit yourself to a small glass (150ml) of pure fruit juice and three fruits per day. Try to avoid bananas (mucus producing) and grapes and mangoes (these are too high in calories).
- Eliminate sugar and refined carbohydrates, i.e., cakes, biscuits, chocolate, puddings. If you crave something sweet, you can have two teaspoons of honey or maple syrup or palm syrup per day. Do not heat or add honey to very hot drinks – when honey is heated it becomes toxic.
- If you have a strong craving for sweets, have a day off once a week and enjoy a single piece of cake, some chocolate or even some toast.
- Avoid fizzy and commercial drinks – they are too high in sugar and artificial sweeteners. Fizzy drinks are carbonated. Carbonic acid depletes calcium from your gut and system and can remove calcium from your bones. During pregnancy you need all the calcium that you can get.
- Drink 2 litres (3½ pints) of room-temperature water daily. Iced water or iced drinks shock your stomach and the related vagus nerve in your solar plexus. This cold shock affects your main digestive organs and may cause indigestion and bloating due to fermentation in the gut. It may even predispose one to pancreatic malfunction.
- Limit your caffeine intake – caffeine encourages water retention and is associated with a higher risk of miscarriage in the first trimester.
- If possible, follow the Homoeopathic Tissue Salt Programme (see page ??): For the third month this is Calc. Fluor. 6c, Mag. Phos. 6c and Nat. Mur. 6c. Take one of each twice a day all through the month. If you live near a homoeopathic pharmacy they will be able to combine the tissue salts into one tablet for you. Alternatively, these are available from the Jeyarani clinic.
- Remember, you only need 200 extra calories per day during pregnancy.

Physical Preparation: Exercise
Throughout this month:
- Avoid vigorous exercise. If you are used to working out in a gym you can still do 20 minutes on a treadmill but at a medium pace. Avoid weight lifting as your pelvic floor is very soft under the influence of the pregnancy hormones and you may damage them. Please avoid the stepping machine and the

rowing machine they can build up your lower vaginal muscles and make the pushing phase of your delivery much harder.

- Do light exercise for 20 minutes per day – this could be a brisk walk from the shops, getting off the bus a stop early or going for a light swim once a week.
- Ask your partner to give you a General Treatment Massage (page 55–64) and Pelvic Drainage (pages 68–9) at least once a week.
- Avoid saunas and steam rooms at all stages of your pregnancy.
- Sun bathing should be limited to only 15 minutes a day throughout your pregnancy.
- Yoga – should commence only after 12 weeks.
- Avoid deep body massage throughout your pregnancy.

Mental Preparation: Self-hypnosis

- If you haven't started already, start listening to your self-hypnosis tape cassette (either the one you have put together yourself or Dr Motha's pre-recorded one). If you can, first attend some self-hypnosis classes for birth preparation (ideally four classes for both partners). These will give you confidence that you can have a healthy pregnancy and a good birth. Check Appendix C for a list of approved practitioners.
- Test your levels of self-hypnosis with the pinch test and arm drop (see pages 111 and 103).

Week-by-week Progress and Recommended Treatments

Week 9

Recommended Treatment   Reiki or Creative Healing with
                                   Reflexology (60 min.)

If you have no symptoms, Reiki is a supportive treatment that you can receive from conception throughout pregnancy. If you suffer nausea and vomiting, have a Creative Healing treatment, along with some light Reflexology.

Note for Practitioner Week 9

Creative Healing: Abdominal toning (pages 66–8), liver drainage and pancreatic treatment.
Reflexology: Very light, avoiding the uterine area.

Week 10

Your baby is 2.5cm (1in) long. The heart is almost completely developed and is working very well with the circulatory system, which is also almost fully formed. Tiny teeth buds are even appearing in the gums. The facial features can be clearly seen on a scan.

Recommended Treatment   Reiki or Reflexology (60 min.)

Note for Practitioner Week 10

Reiki: For deep relaxation.
Reflexology: Light reflexology to boost energy levels and help overcome the tiredness of pregnancy.

Week 11

Recommended Treatment   Creative Healing (60 min.)

This is a very good time to have a heart treatment. Your blood volume is increasing gradually and this is putting an extra load on your heart, so a heart treatment will tone up the cardiac muscle. It also works on an emotional level and will have a calming influence upon you. The heart treatment is always preceded by 10 minutes of abdominal toning. Moreover, a kidney treatment is appropriate at this stage, as the kidneys have to deal with the extra circulatory load.

Note for Practitioner Week 11

Creative Healing: General Treatment (pages 55–64), 10-minute abdominal toning (pages 66–8), heart treatment, kidney treatment

---

Week 12

Your baby's brain is fully formed and your baby can now feel pain. Thumb sucking is observed even at this stage. Eyelids cover the eyes and remain shut till the seventh month.

Recommended Treatment   Reiki or Reflexology (60 min.)

Note for Practitioner Week 12

As per Week 10

Second Trimester

Month 4 (weeks 13–17)

Physical Preparation: Diet

Throughout this month:

- Start drinking the Herbal Tea (see page 11) daily. If you cannot get hold of all the herbs stipulated, then just make it up using the ones that you can buy.
- Start drinking the Baladi Choornam drink (see pages 11–12) daily. To start with, mix one teaspoon of the Baladi Choornam powder in half a cup of hot goat's milk. Slowly build up the dose to two teaspoons by 16 weeks. Add a teaspoon of maple syrup if you would like to sweeten it. (Note: Waitrose supermarket chain does a good brand of goat's milk that is acceptable in terms of flavour and smell. I also like St Helena's brand of goat's milk.)
- Take your Dhanwantaram, or baby pill (see page 12), along with the goat's milk drink (see above). This pill is specially formulated to strengthen your baby.
- Supplements: Vitamins are important at this stage; remember to take your pre-natal/pregnancy vitamin and mineral supplement. In pregnancy optimum doses of vitamin A are essential. (Note: If you are taking a supplement, limit the Vitamin A to 2000–3000IU a day; alternatively Beta-carotene can be taken up to 8000IU a day, and is usually included in your pre-natal vitamin supplement.) See page 11 for recommended brands.

- Limit yourself to a small glass (150ml) of pure fruit juice and three fruits per day. Please avoid bananas (mucus producing), and grapes and mangoes (they're too high in calories).
- Exclude sugar and refined carbohydrates, i.e. cakes, biscuits, chocolate, puddings. If you crave something sweet, you can have two teaspoons of honey, maple syrup, or palm syrup per day. Remember not to heat or add honey to very hot drinks as it becomes toxic when heated.
- If you have a strong craving for sweets, have a day off once a week and enjoy a piece of cake or some chocolate – or even some toast, if you prefer.
- Avoid fizzy and commercial drinks – they are too high in sugar and artificial sweeteners. Fizzy drinks are carbonated. Carbonic acid depletes calcium from your gut and system and can remove calcium from your bones. During pregnancy you need all the calcium that you can get.
- Exclude wheat from your diet – look for alternatives such as rye bread, corn pasta, barley or oats.
- Limit carbohydrates to one portion per meal – i.e. one small cupful of cooked carbohydrates.
- For every portion of carbohydrates, balance it with three portions of vegetables that are recommended for your body type.
- Drink 2 litres (3½ pints) room-temperature water daily – icy water shocks your gut and leads to indigestion.
- Limit your caffeine intake – caffeine causes water retention.
- If possible, follow the Homoeopathic Tissue Salt Programme (see page 12). For the fourth month this is Calc. Fluor. 6c, Nat. Mur. 6c, Silica 6c – take one of each twice a day all through the month. If you live near a homoeopathic pharmacy they will be able to combine the tissue salts into one tablet for you. Alternatively, these are available from the Jeyarani clinic.
- Remember, you only need 200 extra calories per day during pregnancy.

Physical Preparation: Exercise
Throughout this month:
- Do light exercise for 20 minutes per day. This could be a brisk walk from the shops, getting off the bus a stop early or going for a light swim (recently

there have been concerns about the effects of chlorinated water on pregnant women, as well as reported links to asthma. I would recommend swimming no more than once a week in chlorinated pools; or try to find an ozone-treated pool to swim in instead.)

- Yoga can be introduced. Follow the gentle yoga routine featured on pages 75–83 once a day for 20 minutes – preferably first thing in the morning, or last thing in the evening. It can help with overall stamina and suppleness, particularly in the pelvic region. Remember that the daily practice of yoga for 20 minutes is more valuable than a long class once or twice a week.
- Creative Healing massages.
  - Ask your partner to perform a very light and gentle Abdominal Toning (pages 66–8) and Pelvic Drainage massage (pages 68–9) twice weekly.
  - Ask your partner to perform the General Treatment (pages 55–64) once a week for 20 minutes. This will stabilize your blood pressure and prevent back pain.

Mental Preparation: Self-hypnosis

Throughout this month:

- Listen to your self-hypnosis tape cassette daily if possible. If you can, first attend some self-hypnosis classes. Gentle Birth practitioners offer a course of four classes for both partners.
- Top up classes are also offered as on-going support. This will give you confidence that you can do it. (Check Appendix C at the back of this book for lists of approved classes and practitioners.)

Week-by-week Progress and Recommended Treatments

Week 13

You are now entering the second trimester. Your baby is growing longer and stronger. The muscles are developing. The baby's pancreas has differentiated and continues to develop till the 20th week. Even the rudimentary cells that produce insulin are establishing themselves, so you need to eat sensibly as the baby can put on too much weight too early on in pregnancy if you eat too many carbohydrates. This can lead to a big baby who is more difficult to deliver.

Recommended Treatments   Creative Healing (45 min.)
                                         + Reflexology (30 min.)

Note for Practitioner Week 13

Focus on digestive tune-up

Creative Healing: Abdominal toning (pages 64–6) 10 minutes, liver
drainage 5 minutes, pancreatic treatment 30 minutes

Reflexology: For relaxation. Focus on relaxing the oesophagus, along
with liver drainage and pancreatic stimulation

Week 14

The baby's thyroid gland has been developing gradually from 8 weeks and is
almost fully developed at 14 weeks. The baby's thyroid makes hormones that
are important for its bone development. The Creative Healing thyroid treatment
can be self-administered (see description in Practitioner box below) on a weekly basis to keep up your own thyroid gland function, which slows down in
pregnancy. The thyroid hormone is very important for your energy levels and
efficient metabolism. It is essential for the transport of food substances across
cell membranes and into each cell in your body.

Recommended Treatment   Creative Healing (30 min.)
                                         + Reflexology (30 min.)

Note for Practitioner Week 14

Focus on metabolism and thyroid function.

Creative Healing: General treatment (pages 55–64) 10 minutes. Back
and spine treatment (pages 64–6) 10 minutes. Thyroid treatment: Use
the middle 3 fingers of your right hand and use virgin olive oil for
lubrication. Move your fingers on the skin briskly up and down from
the little hollow (between the collar bones at the base of your neck) to
the middle of your sternum (breast bone). In Creative Healing this is

---

described as double vacuuming. Do this for a total of 7 minutes.
Reflexology: Give a thorough treatment with strong clearing moves over the thyroid area. This will set up good energy flows within the thyroid gland and result in normal thyroid function.

Week 15

The focus of your baby's development this week is the completion of the growth of the adrenal glands.

Recommended Treatments   Creative Healing (30 min.)
                                 + Reflexology (30 min.)

Note for Practitioner Week 15

Creative Healing: Kidney and adrenal treatment (10 min.), plus the General Lymphatic Treatment (pages 55–64) (20 min.) and Thyroid treatment (above) (7 min.)
Reflexology: Avoid the uterine area and focus on the kidney and adrenal areas.

Reflexology note: All through pregnancy it is necessary to constantly clear the layers of congestion on the lymphatic areas that correspond to the thoracic and pelvic lymphatics. The reflexes for these areas are situated at the top of the foot and around the ankle areas and during a routine Reflexology treatment at all stages of pregnancy I perform drainage movements along these areas, alternating between the other areas that I work on. Focus on drainage at this early part of pregnancy and it will prevent ankle oedema from ever developing.

Week 16

Your baby is approximately 14cm (5½ in) long and weighs around 170g (6oz). The facial features are becoming more defined and fine hair on the eyebrows and eyelashes begins to grow. Your baby's sexual identity is emerging as the gonads are beginning to differentiate. Sex is determined at fertilization but the external evidence of sex is seen only after 16 weeks. The baby's muscle system is growing in strength and the baby is very active. However, don't worry if you can't feel the baby as yet – this is probably because the placenta has implanted on the anterior wall of the uterus and as such blankets the movements of the baby at this early stage of pregnancy. When the baby grows bigger than the size of the placenta you will be able to feel your baby's movements clearly.

Recommended Treatment   None – Rest week (see proviso below)

Proviso

If you have been having all the treatments, as described in the preceding section of this book, you can have a week to settle between treatments. However, if you are commencing the programme at 16 weeks, as some mothers do, you should have a combination of Creative Healing (65 min.) and Reflexology (30–50 min.).

Note for Practitioner Week 16 (for mothers starting out)

Creative Healing: General treatment lymphatic drainage (pages 55–64) (20 min.) to control blood pressure and decongest; abdominal toning (pages 66–8) (10 min.), this optimizes abdominal comfort. If there is an irritable area within the uterus, such as a seedling fibroid, abdominal toning with the use of the cooling breeze (page 54) can take away inflammation and calm down the irritable uterus. Liver drainage (5 min.) to optimize digestion and abdominal comfort; heart treatment (15 min.); hiatus hernia treatment (8 min.) to prevent reflux; thyroid treatment (pages 152–3) (7 min.) to improve metabolism and provide more energy.

Light Reflexology: If added to the Creative Healing treatment in order to energize the system, 30 minutes. If it is the only treatment being given, the treatment can last 50 minutes. The whole aim of the treatment is preventative. However, if there are specific complaints such as constipation in early pregnancy, you should work on the colon reflexes. Another useful area to work on is the oesophageal reflex in order to keep the gastro-oesophageal sphincter muscle well toned – this will help prevent reflux oesophagitis and retro-sternal discomfort.

Week 17

Recommended Treatment   Cranio-sacral Therapy or Reiki

In an ideal world it would be wonderful to receive Cranio-sacral treatments throughout your pregnancy but if you are living in an area where there isn't a Cranio-sacral practitioner, you should be able to find a Reiki practitioner. Both treatments have similar hand positions. I have observed that Crano-sacral releases have occurred during a Reiki session.

Month 5 (weeks 18–22)

Physical Preparation: Diet
Throughout this month:
- Drink the Herbal Tea (see page 11) daily. If you cannot get hold of all the herbs stipulated, then just make it up using those that are available.
- Have the Baladi Choornam drink (see pages 11–12) daily. At this stage of your pregnancy take two teaspoons of the Baladi Choornam powder in half a cup of hot goat's milk. Add a teaspoon of maple syrup if you would like to sweeten it. If you are just starting the herbs at this stage, start with one teaspoon and then build up to two teaspoons in a week. Add a teaspoon of maple syrup if you would like to sweeten it. (Note: Waitrose supermarket chain does a good brand of goat's milk that is acceptable in terms of flavour and smell. St Helena's brand of goat's milk is a good second choice.)
- Take the Dhanwantaram, or baby pill (see page 12), along with the goat's milk drink. This pill is specially formulated to strengthen your baby.

- Limit yourself to a small glass (150ml) of pure fruit juice and three fruits per day. Please avoid bananas (mucus-producing) and grapes and mangoes (too high in calories).
- Exclude sugar and refined carbohydrates, i.e., cakes, biscuits, chocolate, puddings. If you crave something sweet, you can have two teaspoons of honey, maple syrup, or palm syrup per day. Remember not to heat or add honey to very hot drinks – when honey is heated it becomes toxic.
- Avoid fizzy and commercial drinks – they are too high in sugar and artificial sweeteners. Fizzy drinks are carbonated. Carbonic acid depletes calcium from your gut and system and can remove calcium from your bones. During pregnancy you need calcium.
- Continue to exclude wheat from your diet – look for alternatives such as rye bread, corn pasta, barley or oats.
- You can, however, enjoy one treat day a week, where you can indulge a small craving for something sweet or 'wheaty' – e.g. a piece of cake, some chocolate or even some toast.
- Limit carbohydrates to one portion per meal.
- For every portion of carbohydrates, balance it with three portions of vegetables.
- Drink 2 litres (3½ pints) of water at room-temperature daily.
- Limit your caffeine intake – caffeine encourages water retention.
- If possible, follow the Homoeopathic Tissue Salt Programme (see page 12). For the fifth month this is Calc. Fluor. 6c, Ferr. Phos. 6c, Silica 6c – take one of each twice a day all through the month. If you live near a homoeopathic pharmacy they will be able to combine the tissue salts into one tablet for you. Alternatively these are available from the Jeyarani clinic.
- Remember, you only need 200 extra calories per day during pregnancy.

Physical Preparation: Exercise and Physical Care
- Now that your bump is showing, start to nourish the skin's collagen by applying Jeyarani anti-stretch mark oil to the tummy, breasts and buttocks daily (Appendix C, page 313).
- Do light exercise for 20 minutes per day – a brisk walk or a light swim (ideally in an ozone-treated pool).

- Do the thyroid treatment on yourself weekly (pages 152–3).
- Follow the gentle yoga routine once a day (see page 75), preferably first thing in the morning, or last thing in the evening.
- Receive the Pelvic Drainage massage (see pages 68–9) and Abdominal toning (pages 64–6) twice weekly from your partner.
- Receive the General Treatment massage (pages 55–64) and the Back and spine treatment (pages 64–6) once a week at home.

Mental Preparation: Self-hypnosis

- Hopefully you will have been on a self-hypnosis and visualization course – if not enrol now. Although it isn't mandatory to attend a self-hypnosis course, most mothers find that being coached by a professional for the first few sessions helps them to settle down with the idea of practising self-hypnosis.
- Listen to your self-hypnosis cassette at least two or three times a week. Use the time to switch off from your daily routine and have a deep rest.
- Begin to practise switching in and out of self-hypnosis several times a day, so that on the day of the labour it comes easily to you. You need only stay in a hypnotic state for one or two minutes at a time – what you're trying to do is perfect the technique. Try to practise in different locations.

Week-by-week Progress and Recommended Treatments

Week 18
Your baby is now 15cm (6in) long and has begun to blink and grasp with its little fingers. More fine hair grows on the head and all over the body.

Recommended Treatments   Creative Healing (45 min.)

                                + Reflexology (30 min.)

As your baby grows bigger, there is changing pressure on your spine, hence the need for the General Treatment and the Back and spine treatment which decongests the muscles. During the Back and spine treatment there is repositioning of the substance between the vertebrae to increase the disc spaces – this specific Creative Healing technique is rather unique, as it prevents compression of nerves and is a preventative measure against back pain. A sciatic treatment eases the nerve as it travels along its path in the buttock, the back of the thigh and down the legs. Apart from preventing sciatica from occurring in the future, this treatment also tones up the nerve distribution to all the pelvic structures that deal with nourishing your baby during pregnancy. It also helps to relax the pelvic muscles for birth.

Note for Practitioner Week 18
Creative Healing: General Treatment (pages 55–64), Back and spine treatment (pages 64–6), sciatic treatment
Reflexology: A complete treatment with emphasis on the sciatic area

---

Week 19
Recommended Treatment   None – Rest Week

Your baby is continuing to grow bigger, so take a rest from treatments. Instead, you need to practise your yoga every day for 20 minutes, as well as take a brisk walk for 30 minutes a day. Swim once or twice this week.

Week 20
Your baby is 30cm (12in) long and weighs 450g (1lb). It can hear and recognize your voice. The little fingers exhibit delicate fingernails. Fingerprints appear and there is hair on the head. An ultrasound scan can pick up your baby's sex now too.
Recommended Treatments   Creative Healing (60 min.) +
                                                      + Reflexology (30 min.)

As the baby gets bigger, it begins to sit heavily on the pelvic floor, so a pelvic drainage treatment for 5 minutes will decongest the pelvic lymphatics and encourage a feeling of lightness within your pelvis.

Note for Practitioner Week 20

Creative Healing: General treatment (pages 55–64) (30 mins.): especially loosening of the lower back and sacro-iliac joints (5 min.). Then pelvic drainage (pages 68–9) (5 min.); abdominal toning (pages 66–8) (5 min.); sciatic treatment (10 min.); liver treatment (5 min.); spleen treatment (5 min.) to improve blood content and encourage strong immune function

Reflexology: General treatment

Week 21

Recommended Treatment   Bowen Treatment (60 min.)

The Bowen technique offers neuro-muscular releases for all the skeletal muscles of the body and as such it is profoundly relaxing. The second half of pregnancy brings with it increasing thoughts about the birth. Bowen begins to relax the pelvis and all the other muscles in your body. Your mind automatically feels the possibility that your pelvic spaces will open up to give birth.

Week 22

Recommended Treatment   Bowen Treatment (60 min.)

Two consecutive Bowen treatments are recommended to seal the effects of the functional changes and realignment of structures within the body.

Molecular physicists propose that the human body is composed of molecules organized within our body as a continuous liquid crystal. This helps messages to flow around rather quickly. Bowen aims to heal the tissue memory within the connective tissue and fascia within the body. The application of Bowen treatments in pregnancy benefits the mother by releasing tight holding patterns within the muscles of the pelvis. This will in turn help the pelvic diameters to relax and widen, and encourage the dilatation of the cervix and the descent of the baby's head into the pelvis. A looser inner space within the pelvis means a more comfortable labour.

Week 23   **None – Rest week**
As your baby is maturing your baby's lungs are, in particular, beginning to differentiate and mature. This is a sign that your baby is becoming viable and able
to sustain life outside your womb. You are very thrilled at the prospect that you
have supported your baby so far and you trust that your body will help your
baby develop healthily all the way to term.

Month 6 (weeks 24–27)

Physical Preparation: Diet and herbs
Throughout this month:
- Drink the Herbal Tea (see page 11) daily. If you cannot get hold of all the
  herbs stipulated, then just make it up using those that are available.
- Have the Baladi Choornam drink (see pages 11–12) daily. At this stage of your
  pregnancy take two teaspoons of the Baladi Choornam powder in half a cup
  of hot goat's milk. Add a teaspoon of maple syrup if you would like to sweet-
  en it. If you are just starting the herbs at this stage, start with one teaspoon and
  then build up to two teaspoons in a week. (Note: Waitrose the supermarket
  chain does a good brand of goat's milk that is acceptable in terms of flavour
  and smell. St Helena's brand of goat's milk is a good second choice.)
- Take the Dhanwantaram, or baby pill (see page 12), along with the goat's
  milk drink. This pill is specially formulated to strengthen your baby.
- Limit yourself to a small glass (150ml) of pure fruit juice and three fruits per
  day. Please avoid bananas (mucus-producing), and grapes and mangoes (too
  high in calories).
- Exclude sugar and refined carbohydrates, i.e., cakes, biscuits, chocolate,
  puddings. If you crave something sweet, you can have two teaspoons of
  honey or maple syrup or palm syrup per day. Remember not to heat or add
  honey to very hot drinks as honey becomes toxic when heated.
- Avoid fizzy and commercial drinks – they are too high in sugar and artificial
  sweeteners. Fizzy drinks are carbonated. Carbonic acid depletes calcium
  from your gut and system and can remove calcium from your bones. During
  pregnancy you need all your calcium.

- This is your last month for enjoying one treat day a week and being allowed to eat something sweet or with wheat in, such as a piece of cake!
- Limit carbohydrates to one portion per meal.
- For every portion of carbohydrates, balance with three portions of vegetables.
- Drink 2 litres (3½ pints) of room-temperature water daily. Avoid icy drinks.
- With the exception of your treat day, wholly exclude wheat from your diet – look for alternatives such as rye bread, corn pasta, barley or oats.
- Limit your caffeine intake – caffeine encourages water retention and exhausts your adrenal reserves of energy.
- If possible, follow the Homoeopathic Tissue Salt Programme (see page ??). For the sixth month this is Calc. Fluor. 6c, Mag. Phos. 6c, Ferr. Phos. 6c (same prescription as for month 2) – take one of each twice a day all through the month. If you live near a homoeopathic pharmacy they will be able to combine the tissue salts into one tablet for you. Alternatively, these are available from the Jeyarani clinic.
- Eat moderately – you only need 200 extra calories per day during pregnancy.

Physical Preparation: Exercise and Physical Care

- Nourish your skin by applying anti-stretch mark oil to the tummy, breasts and buttocks daily.
- Do light exercise for 20 minutes per day – a brisk walk or a light swim in a swimming pool (ideally in an ozone-treated pool).
- Follow the gentle yoga routine for 20 minutes once a day (see page 75).
- Receive the Pelvic Drainage massage (pages 68–9 and Abdominal toning (pages 66–8) thrice weekly from your partner.
- Receive the General Treatment (pages 55–64) and Back and spine treatments (pages 64–6) once a week at least from your partner.

Mental Preparation: Self-hypnosis

- Listen to your self-hypnosis tape cassette, at least thrice weekly.
- Continue to practise self-hypnosis in different locations at different times of day.

Week-by-week Progress and Recommended Treatments

Week 24

Your baby is six months old and is becoming more like a real person. Fine hair called lanugo covers the whole body. A waxy substance called vernix protects the skin; this is really layers of unshed skin. The baby seems to be making breathing movements as the ribs and diaphragm practise for air breathing at birth. In the amniotic sac a little bit of amniotic fluid enters the lung. Babies born at 24 weeks can survive with special care.

Recommended Treatments   Creative Healing (60 min.)

+ Reflexology (30 min.)

Note for Practitioner Week 24

Creative Healing: Aim to loosen up the back and neck muscles and to align the spine with a General treatment (pages 55–64) (10 min.) and a back and spine treatment (pages 64–6) (10 min.); abdominal toning (pages 66–8) (10 min.); pelvic drainage (pages 68–9) (5 min.); sciatic treatment (10 min.) Also recommended – extra drainage for sacrum (5 min.) and thyroid treatment (pages 152–3) (7 min.).

Note: Pancreatic treatment (30 min.) should be applied if there are signs of pancreatic insufficiency i.e. distension of the small intestines with trapped wind, coupled with the pancreatic reflex areas on the feet feeling gritty, painful and nodular.

Reflexology: Emphasis on the thyroid and the pancreatic reflex areas. Note: As we approach 28 weeks we have to keep an eye on the endocrine glands, especially the thyroid and pancreas. It is important to improve the blood supply to the whole of the pancreas, including the cells called the islets of Langerhans that produce insulin. Reflexology and Creative Healing on the pancreatic areas have been shown to prevent gestational diabetes and in most cases even correct it.

Week 25

Your baby is growing rapidly and your whole body is expanding. There are amazing fluid changes within your body and you really do notice your bump!

Recommended Treatment   Cranio-sacral Therapy or Reiki
(60 min.)

Week 26

As your baby grows, you are also growing. It is time to take great care of your metabolism and digestive function. Watch what you eat and take care to prepare food that balances your appetite and satisfies you at the same time. Remember to drink your two litres of water every day.

Recommended Treatments   Creative Healing (60 min.)
+ Reflexology (30 min.)

Note for Practitioner Week 26

Creative Healing: General lymphatic treatment (pages 55–64); abdominal toning (pages 66–8) (10 min.); pancreatic treatment (30 min.); liver treatment (5 min.); spleen treatment (5 min.)

Reflexology: Emphasis should be on the pancreas, intestine and the thyroid areas

---

Week 27

As you approach 28 weeks you know that your baby's lungs are getting more mature and ready for life on the outside of your womb. Be aware that you still need to be very careful about your carbohydrate intake. Being careful this week will set a healthy eating trend for the rest of your pregnancy.

Recommended Treatments   None – Rest Week

Third Trimester

Month 7 (weeks 28–31)

Physical Preparation: Diet

Throughout this month:

- Drink the Herbal Tea (see page 11) daily. If you cannot get hold of all the herbs stipulated, then just make it up using those that are available.
- Have the Baladi Choornam drink (see pages 11–12) daily. Take two teaspoons of the Baladi Choornam powder in half a cup of hot goat's milk. Add a teaspoon of maple syrup if you would like to sweeten it. If you are just starting the herbs at this stage, start with one teaspoon and then build up to two teaspoons in a week. (Note: Waitrose supermarket chain does a good brand of goat's milk that is acceptable in terms of flavour and smell. St Helena's brand of goat's milk is a good second choice.)
- Take the Dhanwantaram, or baby pill (see page 12), along with the goat's milk drink. This pill is specially formulated to strengthen your baby.
- Limit yourself to a small glass (150ml) of pure fruit juice and three fruits per day. Please avoid bananas (mucus-producing) and grapes and mangoes (too high in calories).
- It's time to step up your detoxification. A basic wholefood diet will help you to give birth more easily, so from now on exclude your treats altogether.

- If you crave something sweet, you can have two teaspoons of honey or maple syrup or palm syrup per day. Remember not to add honey to very hot drinks as honey becomes toxic when heated or cooked.
- Avoid fizzy water and commercial fizzy drinks – they are too high in sugar and artificial sweeteners. Fizzy drinks are carbonated. Carbonic acid depletes calcium from your gut and skeletal system and can remove calcium from your bones. During pregnancy you need all the calcium that you can get.
- Continue to exclude wheat from your diet – look for alternatives such as rye bread, corn pasta, barley or oats.
- Limit carbohydrates to one portion per meal.
- For every portion of carbohydrates, balance it with three portions of vegetables.
- Drink 2 litres (3½ pints) of room-temperature water daily.
- Avoid coffee altogether – it makes you rather nervy as it over-stimulates your adrenal gland. In pregnancy you need to calm your excitable qualities in readiness for your birthing process. Also, limit tea to one cup per day – tea also contains caffeine and as well as making you jittery it encourages water retention.
- If possible, follow the Homoeopathic Tissue Salt Programme (see page 12). For this month it is Calc. Fluor. 6c, Mag. Phos. 6c, Nat. Mur. 6c (same prescription as for month three) – take one of each twice a day all through the month. If you live near a homoeopathic pharmacy they will be able to combine the tissue salts into one tablet for you. Alternatively, these are available from the Jeyarani clinic.
- Remember, you only need 200 extra calories per day during pregnancy.

Physical Preparation: Exercise and Physical Care
- Nourish your skin by applying anti-stretch mark oil to the tummy, breasts and buttocks daily.
- Do light exercise for 20 minutes per day – a brisk walk or a light swim (ideally in an ozone-treated pool).
- Follow the gentle yoga routine once a day (see page 75), preferably first thing in the morning, or last thing in the evening.
- Do the thyroid treatment on yourself weekly (pages 152–5).

Mental Preparation: Self-hypnosis

- Listen to your self-hypnosis tape cassette at least every other day. You should be easily able to switch into a hypnotic state and the imagery in the visualizations should be most familiar to you by now. Self-programming is invaluable to help you mentally relax about the birth process while your mind is sending birthing messages to your brain, pituitary gland, uterus, cervix and pelvis.

Week-by-week Progress and Recommended Treatments

Week 28

Your baby is viable! Your baby's lungs have begun to secrete a protein that helps the baby to open the lungs with the first breath. This means your baby is getting ready for life on the outside of your womb.

Recommended Treatments   Creative Healing (55 min.)

                                + Reflexology (30 min.)

At 28 weeks, your pancreas will begin to show signs of being antagonized by the placental hormones and hence both the digestive secretions and the insulin secretions may slow down, so a pancreatic treatment can give it a boost.

Note for Practitioner Week 28

Intention: To balance sugar cravings and metabolism

Creative Healing: General treatment (pages 55–64) (10 min.). We need to focus on loosening up the sacro-iliac ligaments to prepare the pelvis for the easy stretching of the pelvic ligaments when the mother is giving birth and draining the sacrum – therefore pay special attention to the sacrum area (10 min.). At 28 weeks, a pancreatic treatment is needed to speed up the pancreatic secretions (30 min.) Liver drainage (5 min.)

Reflexology: General all-round stimulation for all the systems and for lymphatic drainage (30 min.). Focus on the sciatic areas and the sacro-iliac joint reflexes around the ankle.

Week 29

You've settled into your pregnancy and the birth still seems a long way away, but remember – adhering to the programme faithfully will help you to feel light and energetic all the way through your pregnancy. You feel safe that your baby is growing automatically within your womb. You marvel at how your body is taking care of your baby in so many ways.

Recommended Treatment	Cranio-sacral Therapy or Reiki (60 min.)

Notes for Practitioner Week 29

Cranio-sacral treatment: Unwinding of the fascia helps the internal freedom and mobility of the tissues within the body as the mother moves into the third trimester. It is also good to tune into all the cranial bones, test their mobility and free up any restrictions of movements within the membranous cranial bones themselves.

Reiki: The intentions of the practitioner should be the same as that of a Cranio-sacral therapist (see above).

Week 30

Most mothers see 30 weeks as a milestone. It makes you feel as if you have a nice finite number of weeks ahead of you and it becomes even easier to adhere to the programme because you have the end goal in view – of enjoying a confident birth for you and your baby.

Recommended Treatments	Reflexology + Creative Healing treatment (90–120 min.)

The intention of the treatment at this stage is to make more space for the baby within the pelvis by:

• Maximizing the mobility at all the joints of your pelvis

- Helping the soft tissue, i.e. muscles and fascia, within your pelvis to become softer and softer every day, so that they attain the texture of softly-set jelly during the last few weeks of pregnancy

---

Note for Practitioner Week 30

Reflexology: For 30 minutes, concentrating on lymphatic drainage around the ankles and the thoracic lymphatics. The areas around the para-spinal reflexes also hold the reflexes for the abdominal lymphatics and the chain of lymph nodes that run along the inferior vena cava. Working on these thoroughly will improve gut tone.

Creative Healing: As a gentle birth is the result of a healthy physical body, the following Creative Healing treatments are recommended: General treatment (pages 55–64) (20 min.) – this clears the upper thoracic lymphatics and also normalizes blood pressure, an important consideration in the last 10 weeks of pregnancy. Pay a lot of attention to loosening sacro-iliac ligaments and joints (2 min.)

Heart treatment (15 min.) – as the circulatory demands on the mother's heart are increasing with the growing baby it is important to tone up the heart by giving a heart treatment.

Constipation points (10 min.) – perform even if there is no clinical constipation. This treatment keeps the gut clear and helps to clear the pathways of the sacral nerve plexus as these transmit messages to the cervix to open during labour.

Pancreatic treatment (30 min.) – to be added only if the pancreatic area is nodular on the feet.

Liver treatment (2 min.)

Week 31
Recommended Treatment   Rest Week – but …

If the reflex points for the pancreas on the feet have previously been found to be blocked and nodular it would be wonderful to have a repeat Creative Healing pancreatic treatment for 30 minutes. The therapist will be able to teach your partner to give you regular weekly treatments to clear the pancreas. This will be of great help in keeping your blood sugars down. Also, optimum pancreatic secretions help digest your food thoroughly and prevent fermentation in the gut, reducing bloating and wind.

The pancreatic treatment also has an additional benefit. By ensuring normal blood sugar levels in your bloodstream it means that your baby gets just the necessary nutrition and therefore grows to the optimal foetal size for you.

Reminders: Self-hypnosis and Visualization – If you have already attended Self-hypnosis and Visualization classes then that's great and please go for top-up classes! For those who don't have local classes, do listen to your cassette tape as this will facilitate the changes that we would like to see happen within the pelvis.

Month 8 (weeks 32–36)

Physical Preparation: Diet
Throughout this month:

- Continue to drink your Herbal Tea (see page 11) daily, as it helps tone the uterus.
- Have the Baladi Choornam drink each evening, after supper or before going to bed (it helps to soften the cervix). At this stage you should be adding 2 teaspoons of the powder to a small cup of warm goat's milk. Mix well and drink quickly. If you prefer, mix the powder with natural yogurt. Don't forget to take your 'baby' pill with the drink.
- Limit yourself to a small glass (150ml) of pure fruit juice and three fruits (no bananas, grapes or mangoes) per day.

- Eliminate sugar and refined carbohydrates, i.e., cakes, biscuits, chocolate, puddings. If you crave something sweet, you can have two teaspoons of honey per day.
- Avoid fizzy and commercial drinks – they're too high in sugar and artificial sweeteners.
- Wholly exclude wheat from your diet – look for alternatives such as rye bread, corn pasta, barley or oats.
- Limit carbohydrates to one portion per meal.
- For every portion of carbohydrates, balance it with three portions of vegetables.
- Drink 2 litres (3½ pints) of room-temperature water daily.
- Eliminate caffeine from your diet – caffeine encourages water retention.
- If possible, follow the Homoeopathic Tissue Salt Programme (see page 12). For this month it is Calc. Fluor. 6c, Nat. Mur. 6c, Silica 6c (same prescription as for month four) – take one of each twice a day all through the month. If you live near a homoeopathic pharmacy they will be able to combine the tissue salts into one tablet for you. Alternatively, these are available from the Jeyarani clinic.
- Remember, you only need 200 extra calories per day during pregnancy.

Physical Preparation: Exercise and Physical Care

- In week 36, introduce the Vaginal and Perineal Stretch Massage (see page 69). Perform daily, using the perineal massage oil. Strictly not to be performed before week 36.
- Nourish your skin by applying anti-stretch mark oil to the tummy, breasts and buttocks daily.
- Do light exercise for 20 minutes per day – a brisk walk or a light swim (ideally in an ozone-treated pool).
- Follow the gentle yoga routine once a day (see page 75), preferably first thing in the morning, or last thing in the evening.
- Do the thyroid treatment on yourself weekly (pages 152–3).
- Receive the Pelvic Drainage massage (see pages 68–9) and Abdominal toning (pages 66–8) every other day.
- Receive the General Treatment (pages 55–64) and Back and spine treatment (pages 64–6) twice a week.

Mental Preparation: Self-hypnosis
- Listen to the self-hypnosis tape cassette, daily.
- Talk about your safe place with your partner, and elaborate it over the next few weeks.

Ensure you listen to the Birth Rehearsal visualization (see pages 125–9) on a daily basis. (Note: you can also continue listening to your self-hypnosis tape.) You should also ask your baby to release generous quantities of softening hormones from the placenta to convert your pelvic tissues into the consistency of softly-set jelly and each day tell your pelvic tissues that they are becoming twice as soft as the day before. I have seen this simple conditioning work time and time again!

Week 32
At this stage we recognize another landmark – the lower segment of the uterus begins to grow as it is thinner and stretches easily. The growth of the baby means that the baby's position stabilizes within your womb, with the baby's head dropping down into the lowest part of the uterus. The top of the baby's head begins to nudge against the inner part of the cervix and this encourages the cervix to thin out.

You can encourage optimum foetal positioning within your womb by visualizing your baby settling within your womb with the head down. Imagine the top of your baby's head poised above the inner aspect of your cervix, with the baby's chin tucked down onto its chest.

Recommended Treatment	Bowen + Creative Healing treatment (90 min.)

Note for Practitioner Week 32

The intention at this stage is to encourage optimum foetal positioning. Bowen treatment: A full treatment that includes the pelvic and sacral moves. In mothers whose pelvis appears to be narrow the abdominal-coccyx moves can also be added. The intention is to relax the pelvic muscles and to create more room in the lowest part of the pelvis, thus encouraging the baby to find the most comfortable and optimum position within the uterus, i.e. head down.

Creative Healing: General treatment (pages 55–64) (10 min.); heart treatment (15 min.) – increased circulatory load on the mother's heart necessitates a heart treatment; pancreatic treatment (30 min.) – to normalize pancreatic function and keep the blood sugar levels normal

---

Week 33

Your baby is growing and maturing. It is exciting to know that you can communicate with your baby by merely talking to it telepathically.

Recommended Treatment   Bowen Treatment (60 min.)

Note for Practitioner Week 33

As the due date approaches our thoughts naturally gravitate towards the mechanics of the birth of the baby! At this stage, Bowen therapy releases muscle tension and automatically gives the mother deep physical and mental relaxation. Of specific importance are the cleverly designed pelvis release moves that instantly increase the diameters of the pelvis – a gift towards an easier birth!

Week 34

A gentle reminder – exercise and careful eating pays off during the birthing process.

Recommended Treatment   Bowen Treatment (60 min.)

As a rule we advise two Bowen treatments on consecutive weeks. The intention of this second treatment is to stabilize and enhance the effects of the first treatment. If you are suffering from abdominal bloating and still feel bloated after the Bowen treatment, have a Creative Healing treatment too.

Note for Practitioner Week 34

If there still is abdominal bloating then an additional Creative Healing pancreatic treatment can be given for 30 minutes.

Week 35

By 35 weeks you are well acquainted with your baby and the wonderful changes that your body has undergone so far. You are becoming more confident about your body's ability to give birth.

Recommended Treatment   Creative Healing + Reflexology
                                treatment (90 min.)

Note for Practitioner Week 35

The intention at this stage is to build confidence by performing the Creative Healing schedule as set out below and noting the changes that the mother's body has made to accommodate the baby within the womb. Remember to share observations about the amazing softening effects that the mother's body is already exhibiting.

Creative Healing: General treatment (pages 55–64) (10 min.); upper back (10 min.), middle back (5 min.), loosening sacro-iliac joints and

---

drawing the sacrum (5 min.), creating drainage channels for sacrum (5 min.) then pelvic drainage (pages 68–9) (10 min.); heart treatment (10 min.); pancreatic treatment (20 min.); kidney treatment (5 min.)
Reflexology: 30 minutes

Week 36

This is the week that you begin preparing your lower vagina to be able to stretch comfortably and easily when you are giving birth to your baby. At 36 weeks the placental hormones naturally begin to prepare your vagina and pelvic spaces for birth so really we are merely seeking to enhance what nature already sets into action.

Recommended Treatment   Bowen Treatment +/or
                                         Cranio-sacral Therapy (60 min.)

Note for Practitioner Week 36

The intention is to release tendons and ligaments in and around the pelvic and lower abdomen. Both Cranio-sacral therapy and Bowen Treatment achieve this efficiently.

At this stage you should begin doing the Perineal and Vaginal Stretch Massage (see page 69). This should be done on a daily basis from 36–40 weeks. Remember to begin with a gentle stretch and then build up the strength of your stretch. You will be amazed how quickly you will be able to stretch these muscles quite wide with ease. Your confidence in the inherent elasticity of your lower vaginal muscles will increase by leaps and bounds and you will automatically begin to look forward to the confident birthing of your baby at 40 weeks.

Note: This technique can be performed by yourself, or by your partner. If you are self-stretching then the easiest way to do it is to stand up and lift one leg onto a chair then reach down between your legs *from behind* and do the stretches that way.

Month 9 (weeks 37–40)

Physical Preparation: Diet

Throughout this month:

- Eliminate gluten, as well as wheat, from your diet in these last four weeks. Avoid products such as rye bread and oats.
- Drink your herbal tea daily.
- Have your Baladi Choornam drink and 'baby' pill each evening.
- Limit yourself to a small glass (150ml) of pure fruit juice and three fruits (no bananas, grapes or mangoes) per day.
- Eliminate sugar and refined carbohydrates, i.e., cakes, biscuits, chocolate, puddings. If you crave something sweet, you can have two teaspoons of honey per day.
- Avoid fizzy and commercial drinks – they're too high in sugar and artificial sweeteners.
- Limit carbohydrates to one portion per meal.
- For every portion of carbohydrates, balance it with three portions of vegetables.
- Drink 2 litres (3½ pints) of room-temperature water daily.
- Eliminate caffeine from your diet – caffeine encourages water retention.
- If possible, follow the Homoeopathic Tissue Salt Programme. For this month it is Calc. Fluor. 6c, Ferr. Phos. 6c, Silica 6c (same prescription as for month five) – take one of each twice a day all through the month. If you live near a homoeopathic pharmacy they will be able to combine the tissue salts into one tablet for you. Alternatively, these are available from the Jeyarani clinic.
- Remember, you only need 200 extra calories per day during pregnancy.

Physical Preparation: Exercise and Physical Care

- Perform the Vaginal and Perineal Stretch Massage (see page 69) every day.
- Nourish your skin by applying anti-stretch mark oil to the tummy, breasts and buttocks daily.
- Do light exercise for 20 minutes per day – a brisk walk or a light swim (ideally in an ozone-treated pool).
- Follow the gentle yoga routine once a day (see page 75), preferably first thing

in the morning, or last thing in the evening.

- Do the thyroid treatment weekly (pages 152–3).
- Receive the Pelvic Drainage massage (see pages 68–9) and Abdominal toning (pages 66–8) daily.
- Receive the General Treatment (pages 55–64) and Back and spine treatment (pages 64–6) twice daily.

Mental Preparation: Self-hypnosis

- From week 38, begin daily visualizations of your cervix becoming thinner and wider (see page 116).
- Listen to your Birth Rehearsal tape daily.
- Practise going in and going out of self-hypnosis several times a day. If you are having difficulties doing this, practise using your self-hypnosis tape (pages 95–9).
- Elaborate the details of your safe place with your partner if you want. Practise using trigger words to help take you to your safe place.

Practical note – your hospital bag

You should have your hospital bags packed by week 37. By now you are officially at-term and on standby for the birth. Being packed will help you feel psychologically ready to go and avoids scrabbling around once labour has started. But there can be a flip side – it can make the looming imminence of the birth more of a reality, which may make you feel anxious. However, in my experience, most mothers who follow the programme tell me that they are really looking forward to the birth process. Remember that with your confidence-building programme you are now better equipped for your birth than you would have been without this programme – you have already changed your birthing prospects for the better.

Your hospital bag:

Face flannel – to apply to forehead if necessary

Flip-flops/slippers

Socks – many women get cold feet in labour (I do mean this literally, not metaphorically!)

2 cotton dressing gowns

A few cotton nighties or baggy T-shirts

Disposable panties

Breastfeeding/maternity bras

Breast pads

Maternity pads

Toothbrush and toothpaste

Hair tie and hairbrush

Water spray for face

Camera, film and spare battery

Money – especially coins for the phone (note – you're not allowed to use mobile phones in hospital) and for buying snacks and drinks

Video camera

Your Gentle Birth Method kit bag:

This book!

Jeyarani Labour Tape (see Appendix C, page 313) and/or your Birth Rehearsal Tape.

A large bottle of Bach's Rescue Remedy – take a few drops under the tongue every 15 minutes once contractions become regular.

Pre-mixed massage oil comprising 50ml olive oil, 10 drops lavender, 10 drops rosemary, 4 drops rose or neroli or jasmine.

Clary sage essential oil – 4 drops of this oil should be added to the pre-mixed oil mixture above if the contractions wear off.

Lemon glucose tablets for energy (the lemon tends to reduce any nausea).

Comfortable pillow(s).

Walkman and batteries.

Jeyarani Aromatherapy Labour Massage Oil (Appendix C, page 313).

Flask with warm drinking water, teaspoon and cup. (Do not eat ice cubes or drink iced water. This shocks the important nerve plexuses in the abdomen, pancreas and uterus).

Also, homoeopathic remedies (Jeyarani Homoeopathic Labour Kit):

Aconite 200c – useful if distressed, anxious or fearful before or during labour.

Good if labour is too quick or if pains are extreme.

Arnica 200c – the number one trauma remedy. Encourages healing, controls bleeding, reduces swelling and likelihood of pus formation. Nearly all women benefit from it during labour. Reduces exhaustion and gives 'second wind'. Take routinely after birth to speed recovery and alleviate 'battered and bruised' feeling.

Caulophyllum 200c – use as a single dose in the first stage of labour to establish strong, efficient contractions.

Kali. Carb. 200c – useful in 'backache' labours, where nagging pain is felt in the back, buttocks and thighs.

Note:

• For other Homoeopathic remedies that may be useful to have on board during labour, see Section C, pages 312–13).

• Homoeopathic potencies of remedies used in labour are usually 200c though on occasion a higher dose is often indicated.

• If you are using homoeopathic remedies please do not use essential oils (either in massage mixtures or burners) as the two counteract each other. Instead use a plain base oil such as virgin olive oil for massage.

Week 37

Your baby is growing bigger and is settling into your pelvis.

Do the following visualization and bonding exercise every day, as often as you can – even once every hour! Close your eyes and ask your beautiful baby's head to drop head down into your soft and expanding inner pelvic tissues that resemble the consistency of softly-set jelly.

Recommended Treatments   Creative Healing + Reflexology
                                     Treatment (90 min.)

Note for Practitioner Week 37

Keep up the general momentum of clearing congestion in the lymphatics of the back, neck and pelvis. In addition to the Creative Healing, a

---

thorough Reflexology treatment focusing on lymphatic drainage will help the mother to retain high energy levels throughout the last few weeks of the pregnancy. This will help her to exercise regularly and build up her general levels of stamina. After all giving birth requires a mother to be birthfit!

Creative Healing: General treatment (pages 55–64): upper back (5 min.), lumbar loosening and drainage (5 min.), loosening of sacro-iliac joints (5 min.), creating drainage channels for sacrum (5 min.). Back and spine treatment (pages 64–6) (10 min.); abdominal toning (pages 66–8) (5 min.); pelvic drainage (pages 68–9) (5 min.); sciatic treatment (5 min.).

Reflexology: 30 minutes

Week 38

At week 38 we look forward to the baby's head moulding and dropping deeply down into the pelvis and becoming engaged. This is a natural consequence of the downward longitudinal growth of the baby. The upper limit of your abdomen is the diaphragm and ribs, therefore after 36 weeks your baby can only grow in a downward direction towards the pelvic spaces that you have been visualizing as 'soft and wide' all through your pregnancy. Your home practice of Creative Healing to clear the pelvic lymphatics will prove invaluable in the last few weeks, as it has helped your baby's head to descend into your pelvis. Homoeopathy: start taking Caulophyllum 6c three times a week from 38 weeks to term to initiate softening and thinning of the cervix

Recommended Treatment   Bowen Treatment (60 min.)

A Bowen treatment is highly desirable at this stage of the pregnancy, in particular to relax the pelvic areas and create more space for the baby's head to engage deeply within the pelvis. By visualizing the moulding and stretching of the pelvis that usually happens during labour, you will have encouraged this to happen slowly and naturally from 38 weeks to 40 weeks. This means that there will be a reduction in the total time spent in actual labour (i.e. less mechanical work to be done by the uterus) on the birthing day.

Note for Practitioner Week 38

Perform the core moves of the Bowen treatment with additional pelvic, sacral and coccygeal moves (60 min.).

Note: I have found that the 'coccyx move', done at 38 weeks, can help to engage the baby's head and release spasm within the lower vaginal muscles. This helps enable the baby's head to rotate easily within the pelvis during labour.

Week 39

It is a calming thought that you have done so well and have reached 39 weeks! You feel energetic, and you look forward to seeing your baby face to face. Practice yoga for 20 minutes a day. In particular practise your 'funny walks' (see pages 83–5) for 5 minutes three times a day, every day, to increase your pelvic flexibility. For general stamina-building take a brisk walk or swim for 30 minutes a day. Exercise is the best form of detox!

Remember to keep to the recommended food regime as this will keep your tissues in peak condition for a comfy birthing experience. A clear uterus will contract and relax easily. Moreover, clear muscles and tissues in your pelvis will allow your baby to slip through your flexible and soft pelvis in a comfortable manner.

Recommended Treatment Creative Healing, Reflexology + Bowen Treatment (90 min.)

Note for Practitioner Week 39

Dedicate time to loosening and clearing the lymphatics of the back, neck, lumbar and pelvic areas.

Creative Healing: General treatment (pages 55–64): upper back (5 min.), lumbar loosening and drainage (5 min.); abdominal toning (pages 66–8) (5 min.); pelvic drainage (pages 68–9) (5 min.); sciatic treatment (10 min.).

Reflexology: 30 minutes with emphasis on the pituitary areas, the pelvis lymphatics, uterus, kidney and adrenal areas

Bowen: Perform the pelvic release moves (20 min.)

Week 40
Your baby is fully developed within your womb and is ready for birth. Whenever possible visualize the actual day that you will see your baby face to face. Your thoughts will flow to your baby and this will stimulate a response from your baby. Your baby will begin to initiate the secretions from its own brain and hypothalamus and these, together with secretions from its lungs, stimulate the initiation of the birthing process. It is uncanny how you can make this happen!

Recommended Treatments
Reflexology +/or Bowen Treatment and/or Cranio-sacral Therapy (60 min.)

Note for Practitioner Week 40

Reflexology: There is nothing like a deep all-round reflexology treatment at 40 weeks for stimulating all the energy lines within the body and giving the mother a sense of well-being. I have observed that reflexology at 40 weeks seems to 'still' the mother's energy for a while and then gives her the spurt of energy that is so important and necessary in labour. A 30-minute treatment focusing on lymphatic drainage is indicated.

Bowen: Very useful at 40 weeks because it has a deeply sedating effect on the mind and this helps to melt away any anxiety and promotes the natural initiation of labour. Especially useful is the 'coccyx move' which, when applied at term, can help to initiate labour.

Note: A Cranio-sacral treatment: at 40 weeks this treatment can have a profoundly sedative effect. It also offers specific cranial holds (still points) that can initiate labour.

If You Go Over 40 Weeks Gestation…

Firstly remember that the normal duration of pregnancy is between 38 and 42 weeks of gestation. Treatments that can help to initiate labour are Cranio-sacral therapy, Homoeopathy, Reflexology, and Self-hypnosis and Visualization. Most obstetric units routinely follow up mothers at 41 weeks to check that all is going well and propose a management plan.

SECTION C

Having Your Gentle Birth

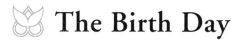 # The Birth Day

Today is the day you meet the baby behind the bump; when you put a face to that little person responsible for all those kicks, rolls and flutters that have kept you enthralled and intrigued; when you get to count all those teeny-tiny fingers and toes – and then count them all over again because you just can't believe how perfect they are.

So how do you feel? Excited? Curious? Thrilled? Calm? Invincible? Well, if you have followed through on your commitment to the programme then chances are that is exactly how you feel. One of the strongest characteristics of a Gentle Birth mother is how much she looks forward to the birth – she can't wait for her show, for her waters to break and for the contractions to start. There's no fear, no regrets, just curiosity about finally getting to experience what she's spent the last nine months preparing for – and the glorious anticipation of meeting her baby face-to-face.

If you feel apprehensive, take encouragement from the fact your baby knows exactly what to do. You could do absolutely nothing at all, except sit in the corner and cry, and you would still deliver your baby (although it would hurt a lot more) because by hook, or by crook, the baby will out. None of us ever knows what our birth experience will be, but you have a rare advantage – preparation. You've trained like an athlete for a marathon and now you are birthfit. By comparison, the other mothers on the labour ward are about to run 24 miles in high heels.

You are on the cusp of one of the greatest achievements of your life, and your body and mind are ready to go. Everything is set for your baby's entry into the world to be as smooth and gentle as possible. What a wonderful gift to give. What a beautiful beginning.

Labour – The first rumblings

- You may have a show up to a week before your baby arrives, so don't get too excited – there may be a few more days to wait.
- If your waters break, ring the hospital. They may ask you to come in for an examination. Once your fore-waters break (the membranes in front of your baby's head) it means the baby is exposed to risk of infection and will have to be delivered within 24 hours. Sometimes the hind-waters rupture and there will be a vaginal leak of amniotic fluid. This happens when there is a rupture of the membranes higher up within the uterus, where they are closely adhered to the wall of the uterus. At term this rupture is usually caused by the fact that the baby has grown to full term and the amniotic sac has thinned out and easily tears as the baby moves around. In this case you will be under observation but there is usually no great urgency to deliver your baby.
- If membranes rupture prematurely, many weeks before your due date, this could be for several reasons that need to be investigated in a proper hospital setting.
- Labour is only considered established when your contractions are coming regularly, every 5 minutes, with each contraction lasting from 30 to 50 seconds. Before then, they may be of varying intervals and strengths or even stop for a while, especially if you relax too much in early labour, for example have a bath too early. Try to hang on till your contractions are well established

before you ring the hospital or midwives (unless your waters have broken).

- If you find the contractions are wearing off, add 4 drops of clary sage oil to your massage mixture and ask your partner to perform a Pelvic Drainage massage (see page 68) and some reflexology on the soft parts of the big toes, (see page 194 in the following section). These should help strengthen contractions.
- If your contractions come on at night, try your best to sleep through them for as long as you can. It is vital to conserve as much energy as possible. Many mothers get very excited when labour starts and rush around but remember, it could be hours before established labour sets in and now, in early labour or pre-labour, is your precious time to rest. Think of yourself as a hibernating bear.
- If you cannot sleep, use some self-hypnosis: listen to the Birth Rehearsal tape, Jeyarani Labour tape, the Self-hypnosis tape or relaxing music to maintain deep muscle relaxation and remain quiet.
- Take some Arnica 200c under your tongue, now (and every 30 minutes during labour) to help minimize swelling within your birthing areas as your contractions push your baby's head firmly into your cervix and pelvic tissues in order to open them.
- Take some Bach Rescue Remedy every 15 minutes to ease the impact of every contraction. This will relax you and help you to manage each contraction, especially if you are a first-time mother.

Once labour is established and the midwives have asked you to go in, get your pre-packed bags and go to the hospital. Ask your partner to drive slowly.

Note to fathers: try to avoid speed bumps!

(If you are having a home birth and your midwives have not arrived already, do ask your partner to call them and say that the contractions have started to speed up!)

Established Labour:
The First Stage

- Reduce stimulus: Dim the lights and keep the door of your room closed to minimize outside noise and disturbance. Switch mobile phones off and make the landline mute!
- As the contractions get stronger, sitting in a warm bath or pool can help take the edge off them, but if you notice the contractions become irregular or weaker, get out and move around.
- Moving around can encourage contractions to become stronger as gravity forces the baby's head onto the cervix, encouraging dilatation.
- If you have a birthing ball, sitting upright with your legs wide can encourage the pelvis to widen and open. Bouncing up and down on it will help gravity to drop your baby's head down even further.
- If you are able to, a squatting position can open the pelvis by 30 per cent.
- Take some Caulophyllum 200c initially and 8 hourly, to help establish strong, efficient contractions.
- If the labour is progressing too fast, take one dose of Aconite 200c – it can help modulate your emotions and help you feel calm.

- If you are experiencing back pain take Nat. Mur. 200c as a single dose.
- If your are exhausted take Kali. Phos. 200c as a single dose.
- Cuprum met. 30c, is useful in labour if there are leg cramps. Take one every 2–3 hours.
- Put on your walkman and listen to the Jeyarani Labour tape (Appendix C, page 313) or your own Birth Rehearsal tape. Visualize your body warming, opening and widening.

The positions that can be adopted in labour
Walking in a darkened environment.

Kneeling on a bed and leaning over an enormous beanbag with your arms draped over the bean bag. Make sure that you kneel on a soft mattress or foam to protect your knees.

Going on all fours on a bed or on a foam mattress placed on the floor. You can even deliver on all fours – this takes the pressure off your pubic area and makes birthing more comfortable.

Sitting in a pool of water once your cervix is more than 5cm dilated. Your time within the pool should be one hour, with a maximum time in the water of two hours. You may need to come out of the water for about half an hour to help you speed up your contractions if they slow down – you can then pop back into the water again. If your pelvis is relaxed you could deliver within an hour of being in the water.

Standing in a warm shower with your partner directing a showerhead of hot water all along your pelvis, sacrum and pubic area. This helps you to cope with the contractions. The warmth of the water will increase blood flow to your pelvic areas and cause your cervix to dilate quickly. Make sure that you can hold firmly onto a handrail within the shower cubicle, as you may feel very sleepy and drift off in between contractions! Your birthing partner should keep a vigilant eye on you. You could have a shower for varying lengths of time, but no more than one hour. While in the shower, a midwife can pop in and listen to your baby's heartbeat every 20 minutes or so with a handheld portable electronic monitor.

Lying on your left side. This helps maximize the blood flow to your uterus and placenta and helps your cervix dilate easily. This position also allows high levels of oxygen into the placenta and keeps your baby well oxygenated.

Don't forget your 'funny walks', e.g. camel or elephant walk, or the figure of eight. These can all help during labour (see pages 83–5).

Standing with the upper half of your body leaning over a raised bed can be very supportive. This gives your partner a chance to massage your back easily and you can still perform the horizontal figure of eight movements with your hips.

Notes to fathers during labour

- Try to control the number of people coming in to the room and asking questions to your partner. See whether you can answer any of their questions on her behalf.
- Ask that they respect the quiet and calm in the birthing room and that they don't do any unnecessary examinations. The more your partner is left to retreat to her safe place, the more quickly the labour will progress.
- Stroke your partner to induce a sense of safety and deep relaxation.
- If she wants you to, talk her through the visualization of her safe place.
- Repeat, like a mantra, the affirmations on encouraging her body to open and relax (see page 101). You should have practised this before the birth.
- Regularly perform some reflexology – every half hour or so – on the soft space in the centre of her big toes (pituitary reflex) for 1–2 minutes at a time to stimulate strong, efficient contractions.
- Regularly perform some Creative Healing treatments to keep her body clear, supple and loose. Creative Healing techniques that are particularly useful during labour are:
  - General Treatment: the Upper Back. Loosening the neck muscles treatment only (page 60).

- General Treatment: the Middle Back (to drain and loosen the lower back) (see page 61).
- General Treatment: the Sacrum. All treatments (see pages 63–4).
- Back and spine treatment (see pages 64–6).
- Abdominal toning (see pages 66–8).
- Pelvic drainage (see pages 68–9).

Father's Tips

- During labour

  There's a lot of pressure on you to be an unfailing support, but don't wear yourself out. Your partner is going to be leaning very heavily on you for mental and physical support and she needs you to be fresh, alert and optimistic, so it is important that you leave the birthing room occasionally – when the mother is relaxed and calm – for some fresh air, a bit of space and a bite to eat. If you tire out, so will she.

- Remember, your partner may not want to be touched or spoken to during contractions, or even throughout the labour. This is absolutely normal and is not something that you or she can predict before the onset of labour. Don't be offended but support her decision. You can still look after her, but in a more passive way, such as making sure the lights are low, the room is not too hot, her feet are warm, and that she is not bothered by countless midwives and junior doctors.

- Treatments to encourage contractions

  Reflexology: There are useful reflex points in the centre of the pads of the big toes (the pituitary reflex points). Apply strong pressure to this area to help the uterine contractions pick up in strength and frequency. 'Vertical' reflexology may be used if the contractions still don't pick up in strength: the mother should stand on a small foot stool with her big toes placed over the edges, you should then reach down and press these points for 3 minutes with pulsing pressure. Repeat at intervals of 15 minutes. I have noticed that this efficiently stimulates the contractions to pick up.

Note: On several occasions, I have done vertical reflexology as described above to keep up the momentum of labour. However, to my surprise, even though the contractions are not noticeably stronger or more frequent, the cervix continues to open to full dilatation. I have even kept up this method of reflexology all the way through the second stage to help the mother deliver – it is very hard work but worth it, as it replaces the need for a syntocinon drip.

Birth Story: Posterior presentation, partner's support and a happy ending – Andrea

My first daughter was only 6 months old when I became pregnant again. My first daughter had come 5 days early, so when I went 10 days over with this pregnancy, I began to think the baby was never going to come out. But then came the tell-tale surge of energy one afternoon, so I ran a bath, lit some candles and enjoyed some quiet time in my safe place.

At 3am I awoke with contractions and by 5am they were 5 minutes apart – so far so good. I felt confident, relaxed and very excited that things were finally happening. At 6am, my midwife arrived. I was 4–5cm dilated but no show or waters broken yet.

My husband went to look after Jade, leaving me happy in my safe place and dealing easily with the contractions. I think I must have been too relaxed because over the next couple of hours, things slowed down. When the contractions fell back to every 8–10 minutes, the midwife got me to move around, to encourage the labour to progress.

This did speed things up. I felt fully in control and pleased that I could remain in a hypnotic state whilst moving around. By 10.30am, the contractions were every 2 minutes, and I took some entonox leaning over a pile of pillows. The midwife checked my progress and to my dismay, I was still only 5cm dilated, although the baby had travelled from ⅔ths engaged to fully engaged. Unfortunately the baby was facing my pubis, rather than my spine, and the discomfort in my back was extreme. I began to find it difficult to stay in control and I think that if I had been in hospital, I would have been asking for an epidural by that stage. All I could think about was how much more I still had to do. A negative mindset was beginning to take over and I knew I was going to lose it if I didn't stay in control.

My husband really was fantastic at this point, encouraging me to stay in control and concentrate on how well I was doing. The urge to push, because of the position of the baby's head, was huge, but I realized I really had to calm down. I managed to focus again and the next two or three contractions brought me to full dilatation. I had gone from 5cm to 10cm in an hour and my baby's head had rotated the right way round to face my sacrum and coccyx.

Finally, my waters broke with a strong contraction and the midwife urged me to push with the next one. It felt fantastic to be able to do something forceful and the head was nearly out on the first contraction. Another three pushes and we had our beautiful baby girl. It was 11.47am, an hour and a quarter after labour was fully established. She weighed 8lb 9oz and I needed only one cosmetic stitch internally.

Established Labour: The Second Stage

- The pushing can take longer than mothers realize but don't become despondent if it takes more than 10 minutes! Most of my mothers who have practised the vaginal stretch technique have a short 20-minute pushing stage. However, if you have a baby who is a bit big for your pelvis and if your baby's head has to undergo considerable moulding to come through, the pushing stage can go on for two hours. Your baby is now only perhaps a fingertip away from being born – be patient.
- Whilst you must remain patient, do not stay too relaxed at this stage. A little adrenalin can help you find the burst of energy and power you need to push the baby out.
- If you feel an almighty urge to 'bear down', before the midwife says you are ready, taking quick shallow breaths can help you resist the urge to push.
- If you use a squatting position, sit in a supported squat as it creates more space within your pelvis for birth. Squatting too deeply in the pushing stage might stretch the perineum too much and cause you to tear more easily.
- For delivery, squatting in a pool of water can be very supportive as the water takes more of the weight off your legs.

- Only push with the contractions.
- Once the baby's head starts to come out, maintain your focus on your baby's head, gently stretching your vagina to its fullest elasticity. Your dedication to pre-birth stretch exercises will help greatly towards your baby's head not slipping back into your vagina between contractions.
- It is wonderful to reach down and touch the baby's head. Many mothers find this very encouraging and an emotional reward for all their efforts. One of my mothers, Janey Lee Grace (read her story on page 200), described her baby as feeling like a fuzzy, little duckling, which I thought was very sweet.
- When your baby's head is born, it is very important to focus on relaxation and wait for the next contraction before pushing the rest of your baby out.

Established Labour: The Third Stage

- Do not cut the umbilical cord until it has stopped pulsating. Your baby will have started to breathe through its nose and mouth as soon as its skin hit the cooler air in the room. After this your baby does not need the umbilical cord for oxygen anymore, but the surge of endorphins that come immediately after the birth are exchanged between mother and baby through the cord and this makes both mother and baby feel mutually exhilarated and can help with deep bonding.

- Ideally, the placenta should be naturally expelled from the body. Contractions (milder than those during labour) will usually push it out within half an hour of delivery. To help expel the placenta, use Sabina 30c as a single dose. If there is increased bleeding, use Secale 30c as a single dose. If there is profuse bleeding use a single dose of Phosphorus 200c.

- After delivery if you get 'the shakes' with nervous exhaustion take Kali. Phos. 30c as a single dose.

- If you are exhausted and also have had excessive bleeding or fluid loss, i.e. vomiting or diarrhoea, take China 30c as a single dose.

Birth Story: Long labour – Janey Lee Grace (Radio 2 presenter)

In May 1999, when my son Sonny was about 7 months old, I started to feel really quite ill. I had no energy and was dizzy and exhausted, which was very unusual for me. I put it down to the fact that I was working and still breast-feeding.

I've always been into alternative treatments so I went to see my homoeopath who told me to eat more healthily and continue to take my B vitamins. I also found I'd gone off coffee and alcohol. It was as if my body was forcing me to detoxify.

I was about to start as co-host on *Steve Wright in the Afternoon* on Radio 2, and my partner had bought me a big bunch of flowers to celebrate. The smell of the lilies made me feel quite sick and I suddenly remembered being pregnant with Sonny, when I couldn't stand the smell of flowers, scented candles or any of my favourite perfumes. Suddenly it all made sense.

I took a pregnancy test but didn't really have to look at the blue line. I just knew I was pregnant. I had a scan, which determined that I was already 13-weeks pregnant. My due date was January 10, 2000 – I was going to have a Millennium baby.

I'd only been working with Steve for about a week when I told him I was pregnant. He was delighted for me and very keen to tell the nation. I had loads of letters and calls to congratulate me. It saved me a lot of phone calls, as people I hadn't spoken to in ages rang up and said 'I heard on the radio you're pregnant.'

The pregnancy went well. The dizziness and tiredness soon passed and I got my energy back. Regular reflexology and massage helped keep my body – and pelvic region in particular – free of congestion. I took all my herbs and listened to the visualization tape every day. It was so relaxing I often fell asleep listening to it, but I'm sure the positive messages still got through.

The New Year passed and around 6pm on January 12th, I had a 'show' and at about 1am we headed off to hospital.

A lot of my friends had said 'oh second babies just fall out'. Well, mine didn't! I was only 3cm dilated when I arrived at the hospital and the baby's head hadn't engaged yet, so I knew it would take some hard work to get everything moving.

It was a long first stage – about ten hours. The dilation was happening slowly, but the baby's head was still high – in no way did he want to get engaged. I wore my walkman and listened to the visualization labour tape. I paced the corridor, stopping to lean over a windowsill every so often to have a contraction, whilst imagining my cervix opening up.

After a few hours, I got into the birthing pool, which provided wonderful pain relief, but unfortunately I couldn't stay in the water throughout because I had to be examined regularly.

I was offered gas and air, but felt sure it would make me auseous, so declined. After I'd been on the go for 8 hours though, one of the midwives gave me a glucose tablet – I'd forgotten how much energy I was using up.

I desperately didn't want intervention and my biggest fear was I was enduring all of this, only to have to have a forceps to bring the baby's head down, or worse still, an emergency Caesarean.

Back in the pool, we lit some candles and put some aroma-therapy oil in the burner. The midwife massaged my shoulders and back, and gave me a Reiki treatment, while Gowri gave me cranial-massage, continuing to stimulate the points that help to dilate the cervix. Throughout the proceedings, she continued to talk to me, helping me to visualize my baby getting ready to be born. She told me that I had plenty of strength to continue and that I could do it – I believed her. She inspired me totally.

After what seemed like weeks (but was actually nine hours), something seemed to change. Part of the waters surrounding the baby had already broken but all of a sudden, the rest broke in a gush. I became very tearful and desperate and felt the urge to push.

I was half-sitting, half-squatting in the pool, and it only took a few pushes for the head to crown. The midwife asked me if I wanted to guide the baby's head out myself. I put my hand down and it was wonderful – it felt like a little duckling!

It's hard to describe the feeling when he floated up to me: I just saw his blue eyes and lots of silvery blond hair. Euphoric is the word, I suppose. I hadn't even asked if my baby was a boy or a girl.

I put my new son to my breast and he suckled immediately – he seemed to know just what to do. We waited for the cord to stop pulsating before Simon cut it, and then I gave one more big push and out came the placenta.

Then it was time for refreshment and I can honestly say it was the best cup of Earl Grey I've ever tasted. The obstetrician examined me and although the baby was quite big, at 8lb 4oz, with a big head circumference, I had no tears – the massage oil had worked. Simon then rang Steve Wright, who was in the middle of his show. He congratulated us on air, and that was how most of my friends found out that I'd had a baby boy.

I believe the preparation I'd done during pregnancy really helped, and there's no doubt that the reflexology during pregnancy and the labour really played a part. I definitely think that without the vaginal oil, I would have needed stitches. I'm also told that my recovery was remarkably quick – Buddy Jackson was born at 2.40pm on Friday afternoon and the next morning we were out having cappuccinos in St John's Wood high street.

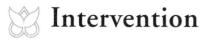 # Intervention

If your labour has been going on for eight or more hours and dilatation is very slow or inconsistent, then I do advise considering forms of pain relief, such as an epidural. You may think this is inconsistent with the non-interventionist aims of this programme, but I am a doctor and I have seen mothers who, even with preparation, have babies who are a bit too big for them to deliver without assistance, and I do believe in medical intervention when needed – just not automatically as a front-line treatment.

The difficulty in accepting medical intervention once you have followed a birth preparation programme is that it is easy to regard any kind of help as failure on your behalf. But this just isn't the case. However much you condition yourself for birth, there are never any guarantees that events will unfold as hoped. The birth rehearsals we have visualized are hypothetical scenarios that occur when there are no presenting problems, but if difficulties do arise, the best thing you can do for yourself and your baby is to be open-minded and flexible – rigidly keeping to your 'birth plan' can sometimes be detrimental to your well-being and that of your baby. The technology and expertise in medical obstetrics is there to help you and you should use it if you need it.

Success is delivering a healthy baby, not 'winning' the birth challenge. There are no medals for going through labour without pain relief and I firmly believe that an epidural, or other such method of analgesia, is preferable – and more gentle – than a long, protracted and tortuous birth that leaves both mother and baby exhausted and traumatized. The underlying principle of the Gentle Birth Method is that you do what's best for your baby and you – and sometimes that does mean medical intervention.

If you do decide upon intervention, I recommend the following pain relief (in chronological order):

- Entonox (gas and air)
- Low-dose epidural, also known as the 'mobile epidural'. Please note this is a misnomer – you cannot freely 'walk around with it' because you are attached to the drip stand and monitors. The low dose means that it uses drugs that maximize the anaesthetic effect while allowing you to feel your legs and, with help, walk to the loo when you are detached from the monitors or drips. When you are fully dilated and ready to deliver, the epidural dose is withheld and this will enable you to feel your contractions and push your baby out with the contractions.

I do not recommend Pethidine, as this can cross over the placenta and make the baby drowsy. I am also not a fan of TENS machines as I am suspicious of anything which interferes with the neurological pathways. After all, our bodies are electrical circuits and I do not think foreign currents should be applied to them. Some Naturopaths take this so far as to tell people to avoid wearing battery-powered watches and choose a kinetic design instead. Certainly, you might like to take your watch off when labour starts – it will also stop you clock-watching the moment your contractions start.

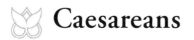 # Caesareans

In 2001, 9.8 per cent of Gentle Birth Method first-time mothers required a Caesarean. This compares favourably with the national overall average of 25 per cent (it is higher for first-time mothers, at 40 per cent). While I hope to bring my percentage rate down yet further, I do think it is encouragingly low – and also realistic. There will always be some mothers who need medical intervention to give birth to their babies, therefore I don't think there will be a time when 100 per cent of mothers receive the birth they want. So if you become one of this 10 per cent, please take heart that we are all subject to Nature's whims and cannot control everything that happens to us. There will always be an element of the unknown – the best we can ever do is try to create the best conditions for achieving what we want.

If you do have a Caesarean, I hope you will still have a rightful sense of achievement for the way you nurtured your baby in the womb and made that environment as calm and soothing as possible. At the very least, you should come away from the programme having enjoyed a blooming, asymptomatic pregnancy during which you bonded deeply with your baby and started your long journey down the road together as a family. Be comforted too, that the incidence of post-natal depression is very low indeed in my mothers. Also, because you've controlled your diet, your figure shouldn't be very different to how it was pre-pregnancy, even soon after having your baby.

And remember, there's always a next time. You have an 80 per cent chance of a vaginal delivery following a Caesarean section, and I hope you will still have faith to be a Gentle Birth mother.

Here are some accounts from a few of my mothers who did have to have caesareans.

Case History: Sarah

I started Dr Motha's programme three weeks into my second pregnancy. I followed all aspects of the programme, except the exercise and cutting out sugar.

Two weeks before Marcus was born, Gowri and I felt something could go wrong and we dealt with the possibility of it openly, so that I was prepared. Although I'm only 5ft 2in, the baby was large and lying in the posterior position. Despite being fully dilated, I was unable to deliver and 9lbs 2oz Marcus was delivered by emergency Caesarean.

Gowri and I were both disappointed at the outcome, but I wasn't disappointed in Gowri. I had a good pregnancy and felt very well after the birth. I would certainly birth with Gowri again, and next time around I'd cut out sugar and would definitely exercise.

Case History: Karen

It was week 40 and I was booked in for a routine hospital check, the day after my due date. All week, I had felt that labour was not imminent, so when the midwife diagnosed the baby as breech, things made sense to me. The hospital did a scan to check the baby's position, in order to see if a manual turn would be possible, but his neck was twisted so that he was facing outwards, which made it dangerous. He was also found to be what is called 'footling' breech which increased my risk of cord prolapse (the cord becoming trapped in the cervix if my waters broke) from 10 per cent to 25 per cent. The doctors said they could not afford for me to go into labour and that I had no choice but to have a Caesarean.

I was terrified and absolutely devastated, and called Gowri as soon as I had told my husband. Gowri came to see me, to do a visualization of the baby turning and to show me how to use Moxa sticks, which can help the baby to turn. These are used in Chinese medicine and if used between weeks 32 and 36 have a 70 per cent success rate. It didn't look good though. The baby was big and with his awkward position, we couldn't really see him turning, even if he wanted to.

I was booked in for an elective Caesarean two days later but my husband and I set to work with the Moxa sticks, using them twice a day, and I spent a lot of time lying on the sofa willing the baby to turn.

On the day of the operation, I woke at 6am to take an antacid pill that the consultant had told me to take before coming into hospital. My husband also had a last ditch attempt with the Moxa sticks. At 6.20am, I felt a strange sensation and thought the baby was turning. The feelings became more and more regular, from every twenty minutes to every ten, and by the time we went to hospital at 8am, they were coming regularly every 5 minutes and lasting for 1 minute each. I had spontaneously gone into labour!

I told the nurse when we booked into the ward that I was in labour but I think my apparent comfort and ability to easily move about made her think I was exaggerating – or just hopeful. She hooked me up to the monitor and when she came back an hour later, the contractions were every three minutes. She couldn't believe it. I lay on the bed, practising my deep muscle relaxation and retreating to my safe place – I was delighted at how easily it came to me – whilst theatre was prepared. I had now become an emergency Caesarean as everything was happening so fast – I was 6cm dilated and they still wouldn't let me deliver naturally.

I walked myself to theatre – albeit slowly – savouring every single one of my contractions. Having committed myself to the programme throughout my pregnancy, I had been so upset that I was going to be denied my labour. It sounds crazy but I really wanted it – I just couldn't wait for contractions to start. I was scared that having an operation to deliver my baby would be clinical and unemotional and I thought that by not 'working' for my baby, it would affect the bonding process.

But in the end, the birth was beautiful. Very intimate and controlled, and I was so thrilled that I had my labour after all. I shall definitely do the programme with my next pregnancy and, fingers crossed, I am fully intending to have a vaginal birth.

Letters

I have received hundreds and hundreds of letters from the mothers who have enjoyed Gentle Births and, of course, it is impossible to include them all. However, I have selected a small core for you to read, to show you the experiences of some of the mothers who have gone before you. You'll find the letters in Appendix B on page 303.

Post-natal Care

Congratulations! You're a mummy, a daddy, a family. You're discovering the joys of possetting, winding, hopefully breastfeeding, acclimatizing to 24-hour living and a huge psychological shift in which your world is suddenly not about you. For the next few weeks, at least, your baby's the boss.

There's so much to learn in the ensuing weeks and months. You're on probably the steepest learning curve of your life and you're rapidly becoming an expert on your baby. Adrenalin will really help you get through the first few weeks – many mothers and fathers claim not to be remotely exhausted on just three hours sleep a night in the first month – but once the initial euphoria dissipates, the going can get tough. So be on the lookout. As a Gentle Birth Method parent you already know that prevention is better than cure. Here are some tips for making the most of the early months.

Rest

Don't wear yourself out. In India, following the Ayurvedic tradition, mothers spend the first 40 days resting in their mother's home and are massaged every day to restore muscle tone and skin elasticity. It sounds utterly luxurious to western cultures, but actually this is a very practical tradition. Mother and baby are allowed to rest together, bond deeply, and establish breast-feeding. It may not be practical for you to follow this ritual, but at the very least, sleep when your baby does and forget about the housework and cooking. (I recommend my mothers prepare some frozen meals before the birth – these can then be easily defrosted and re-heated in the first few weeks.)

Homoeopathic remedies
Take the following remedies daily for the first five days:
- Arnica 30c, Bellis perennis 30c and Hypericum 30c at the same time, three times a day. These reduce pain and swelling.
- Calendula 30c: Take this an hour after the above combination if you have had a Caesarean, or a vaginal/perineal tear – it helps speed the healing of cuts and wounds.
- Add 15 drops of Mother Tincture Hypericum to 7cm (3in) of water in a glass and, using small cotton pads, apply this to the bruised areas.
- Chamomilla 30c: This is good for the after-pains of labour (caused by the uterus contracting down). Take twice a day.
- Kali. Phos. 30c can help with exhaustion or broken sleep. Take a single dose.

Massage
- Have a general full-body massage every day for the first 10 days after birth. Having a postnatal massage with Rose Otto in a two per cent solution has been found to lift the mother's mood and prevent baby blues. It can be performed by your partner or a therapist over as much of your body as possible – neck, back, abdomen, arms and legs. Creative Healing therapists will also incorporate the heart treatment, abdominal toning, pelvic drainage and the sciatic treatment.

Reflexology
- If possible, have a reflexology treatment once a week for the first 12 weeks. After the birth, reflexology can help to restore your sleep patterns, will help with your milk let-down if you are breastfeeding, and is deeply calming. It also helps the uterus to contract and return to its normal size and tone.

Bowen Treatment

- This will help to re-align your pelvis after the birth and boost your general return to recovery. Bowen can also be given to your baby to relieve colic or vomiting. It is so gentle it can be given from day one, if you like.

Case History: Persistent vomiting – Kirsty, aged 6 weeks

Kirsty was vomiting after every feed and was not absorbing her milk. She had been thoroughly checked by the paediatrician and nothing was found to be wrong. However, Kirsty was agitated and her mother was anxious and worried. Immediately after the Bowen treatment, Kirsty calmed down and began to stretch, before falling asleep. Her mother rang the next day to say she had fed Kirsty for the first time without the baby vomiting afterwards and she seemed more settled. Since then she has had no recurrence of the problem.

Creative Healing

- I recommend a general abdominal toning treatment within a week after the birth to evenly distribute the energy within the abdominal organs. This can be done at home (see page 67). An instructional DVD can also be obtained from us (see page 314 for details). Alternatively, see a Creative healer (consult Appendix C on pages 309–11).
- I also recommend a pelvic drainage treatment to help resolve any pelvic oedema that may occur. Also, taking the heat off the lower abdomen and bladder area can make passing water more comfortable after birth. This can be done at home by your birth partner (see page 68). This technique can be seen on the instructional Creative Healing DVD, which can be obtained from us. Alternatively, see a Creative healer.
- It is important that after the birth, the uterus, cervix and neck area of the bladder are toned, lifted and restored to their original position – this helps prevent uterine prolapse and stress incontinence. Ideally, this should be

done two weeks after birth and repeated at 4 weeks and then 6 weeks post-natally. Visit a Creative healer for this specific technique.

- I also recommend a heart treatment after birth, as it has been placed under a lot of strain, and this is a good boost for your general health levels. This needs to be done by a Creative healer.
- In the unlikely event of haemorrhoids (piles) a specific Creative Healing treatment over the coccyx and sacral area is very efficient in reducing them. The technique involves drawing up a skin fold using the flats of your thumbs. Place each thumb horizontally on either side of your coccyx about a centimetre width apart, using virgin olive oil as a lubricant, push the fold of skin directly upwards with firm pressure to the top of the sacrum. This is done repeatedly for about 10 minutes per day. This treatment can be done immediately after birth, or as soon as they are noticed. This technique can also be seen on the Creative Healing DVD. For other helpful hints on how to manage piles, please see page 261 in Section D.

Reiki

- If you feel very tired after the birth, a hands-on Reiki session will be deeply relaxing for you. If possible, have a session immediately after the birth and then weekly, or as often as you can.

Cranio-sacral therapy for mother and baby

Even in problem-free births, the pressure of the baby's head on the mother's pelvic floor during contractions commonly creates compressions to the base of the baby's skull. In addition, during birth, the mother gets into positions that she wouldn't normally assume and her pelvic tissues are pressed by the emerging baby. As a result, the connective tissue between muscles and bones may become stretched and disturbed by the birth, leading to the following complaints.

- Baby: Problems in the baby, like colic, sucking problems and respiratory difficulties, may be due to compressions and strains arising from the birth. These can become bigger problems later in life – such as migraines, sinusitis, depression, spinal and pelvic pain.

- Mother: Internal bruising following the birth may lead to scar tissue, which can later manifest as pelvic pain. If the mother has had a very prolonged pushing phase the lower vertebral ligaments may also be sprained and, if left untreated, this may give rise to chronic lower back pain.
- Ideally, I recommend an early treatment for mother and baby in the first few weeks after the birth and, if possible, regular follow-ups at weekly or fortnightly intervals.

Clinical Notes: Post-natal pelvic pain – Sally

Sally had not been one of my mothers during her pregnancy, but her labour had been long and arduous – a managed affair with syntocinon induction, two epidural attempts and a ventouse delivery with strong pulling of the baby out of the pelvis.

The epidural had numbed Sally's usual protective reflexes and put an abnormal stress on the ligaments and muscles of her pelvis. She presented seven days after the birth, barely walking, with both legs widely abducted in an exaggerated gait.

On local examination, in addition to the sprained lumbar muscles, she had a marked scoliosis (curvature of the spine) that she said had existed from childhood.

I gave her one 45-minute Creative Healing session, starting with the general lymphatic treatment on the back. I found the shoulder muscles very tight and rock hard in consistency so I took the heat away using the cooling breeze method (a Creative Healing technique). I then decongested the whole of the lower back to clear away the oedema that is usually associated with acute tissue trauma. I applied a Creative Healing sciatic treatment and treated both the upper and lower sciatic nerve distribution areas.

As the Bowen technique is very good for acute conditions, I then applied a 20-minute core integration move that worked on her back, respiratory muscles, front and back of the thighs, pelvis and coccyx.

I also advised her to wean herself off her prescribed painkillers (NSAIDs) and to replace these with homoeopathic Arnica 200c three times a day; and 4 drops of Rescue Remedy three times a day for one week.

After one week, Sally walked in with a much better gait and said that she was feeling a lot better. She was off her painkillers and was breastfeeding satisfactorily. She had two more 30-minute treatments of Creative Healing and Bowen, after which she felt restored.

SECTION D

A–Z Guide to Symptoms and Potential Problems in Each Trimester

Think of pregnancy as a package deal – your baby is the destination, but there are all sorts of inclusive extras along the way, such as heartburn, varicose veins and, of course, the fabled morning sickness. Most are unpleasant and ideally avoided, but some mothers learn to love their side-effects. Why? Well, pregnancy usually announces itself through symptoms and in that limbo period while you're waiting for your baby bump to spring forth or longing for the first kick, symptoms are there to tell you the pregnancy is still continuing and progressing.

However, even the most enthusiastic mother can tire of morning sickness whilst battling to work in the rush hour, so it's little wonder side-effects have got such a bad name. But there is a lot you can do to help yourself either eradicate or dramatically reduce your pregnancy symptoms. This section looks at the side-effects common in each trimester of pregnancy, the reasons why they're happening and how you can go about alleviating or eliminating them. We also examine some of the complications that can occur, particularly in the final trimester, such as eclampsia or a breech presentation, and what you can do if your baby is overdue.

The First Trimester

Your body in the first three months

It's rather unfair that the enormous changes happening in your body in the first three months are all unseen, because it really is very impressive. Your physiology changes, with your kidneys, liver and heart all enlarging and your blood volume increasing by 30 per cent (although your blood pressure remains the same). Then the hormones kick in, with more than sixteen times the amount of progesterone found in a normal menstrual cycle, and more than 300 times the normal amount of oestrogen. All this is happening to facilitate organo-genesis, whereby the baby's templates (central nervous system, cardio-vascular, skeletal systems and so on) are created. A new life is being created, your own mini miracle, and you're doing it in your sleep. Who wouldn't want some applause?

Your baby in the first three months

Your baby undertakes a mammoth journey of growth and development during the first trimester – and it's taking all the nutrients, hormones and energy it needs from your body.

By the time you miss your first period, your fertilized egg (embryo) looks like a ball of cells and at this stage has already settled in your uterus. Part of this ball of cells attaches onto the lining of your uterus and forms little root-like structures called chorionic villi. These will eventually become the placenta. Within the ball of cells a small amniotic-fluid-filled sac develops and your baby appears as a little line of cells that differentiates to form a fully-formed baby.

The embryo starts off as three different layers of cells. The neural tube – which fosters the spinal cord, nervous system, brain and backbone – develops in the top layer. The heart and circulatory system appear in the middle layer and the last layer grows the lungs and intestines. By the time you are seven weeks pregnant, your embryo already has a pumping heart and is making its first movements – stretching, kicking and waving.

The embryo is officially considered a foetus by week 9, as its embryonic tail has gone, and it is growing downy hair and fingernails. By the end of the trimester – at 12 weeks – it has articulated limbs (defined ankles, elbows, wrists, knees) and fully formed and functioning vital organs – brain, lungs, kidneys and liver. Your foetus is probably around 6cm long now and with its critical development over, all that remains is for the baby to grow and lay down fat in order to survive outside the womb. And you wonder why you feel so tired.

Trimester One: A–Z Guide

Abdominal Pain

What is it?: A sharp or pulsing pain in the abdominal cavity.

What causes it?: The commonest cause is wind. In the early part of pregnancy, it is due to the increased progesterone in circulation. Intestinal mobility and digestion can slow down, resulting in trapped wind.

Other causes can be cystitis and stretching pains due to the sudden growth of the round ligament in the pelvis, causing tendinitis. Bear in mind that abdominal pain can also indicate more serious conditions, such as appendicitis or indeed be an early sign of miscarriage.

Important note:
- If there is even just a small amount of spotting of blood vaginally, see your doctor immediately. You will need an early foetal scan to check that all is well with your baby and to make sure that your baby has implanted within your uterus. The doctor will also rule out any serious abdominal conditions. Note: Take a urine sample in a sterile pot to your GP to test for urinary infection.

How can it be alleviated?:
- Rest is the first option.
- Peppermint tea will release trapped wind. (Note: peppermint counteracts the action of homoeopathic remedies so take this *or* a homoeopathic remedy.)
- Creative Healing: The whole abdominal cavity can be eased by general abdominal toning (see pages 67–8) for 10 minutes. The Creative Healing instructional DVD shows this technique (see Appendix C, page 314 for details). Alternatively see a Creative Healer.
- Homoeopathic remedies:
  - For colicky abdominal pain that is relieved by a warm compress, take Mag. Phos. 30c. Dissolve one dose in a third of a glass of lukewarm water and sip and stir the glass as you go along (stirring makes the remedy more potent).

- If the pain is caused by exaggerated Braxton-Hicks, the best remedy is Cimifuga 6c three to four times a day. If the pain is relieved by doubling over and hard pressure, and you feel irritable, try Colocynthis 30c as a single dose.

Anaemia

What is it?: The reduction of haemoglobin (red blood cells) in the blood, commonly manifested as tiredness, and often diagnosed by the GP by a routine blood test.

What causes it?: It is usually due to nutritional deficiencies of iron, folate or vitamin B12 – but in pregnancy can also be ascribed to haemodilution, which occurs when the increase of blood volume leads to dilution to blood content.

How can it be alleviated?:

- Iron deficiency can be resolved with iron tablets. Floradix is a herbal iron tonic and as a natural source of iron it is preferable to pharmacological-grade iron supplements, which can cause constipation.
- Folate deficiency can be resolved with oral folic or folinic acid tablets.
- Improve your diet. Eat more chicken, lamb and moderate quantities of dark leafy green vegetables such as broccoli and cabbage. Beware though, too much of these will cause wind!
- Avoid tea as tannic acid interferes with efficient iron absorption.
- Drink nettle tea and a ⅓ of a glass of orange juice each day as these help with the absorption of vitamin C and iron.
- Dried fruits such as apricots are very high in iron, but are also high in sugar, so limit the amount you take to about 3–5 pieces a day.
- Avoid milk with a protein meal as it prohibits absorption of iron by up to 50 per cent.
- Cook in an iron pan.
- Homoeopathic remedies:
  - For iron deficiency take Ferr. Phos. 6c and Ferr. Met. 6c together, four times a day, for several days
  - Folic acidum 6c is a recommended homoeopathic remedy for folic acid deficiency

Anxiety

What is it?: Feeling uncharacteristically tearful, overwhelmed or stressed by everyday concerns.

What causes it?: Even if you are joyous about being pregnant you may still suffer anxiety. This can be for a number of reasons including: you can't stop thinking about the changes in lifestyle you will have to make to accommodate your new baby; if you don't feel at ease in your home environment; if you have a very stressful job you may find yourself getting anxious and fearful about how you will cope with motherhood; sometimes even a loving father may be away at work most of the time and this can lead to feelings of isolation and anxiety.

How can it be alleviated?:

- If possible, see a counsellor – they will help you to voice your concerns and assist with lifestyle modifications. At the very least, share your concerns with your partner and close friends.
- I recommend some Bach flower remedies – Walnut is good for big changes in life, Aspen helps release unconscious anxieties, and Mimulus is indicated for specific fears and worries. Take 4 drops of one or all of these in a glass of spring water and sip slowly.
- Exercise, in the form of a brisk walk, releases endorphins and is an automatic mood elevator.
- Homoeopathic remedies (for all, the dose is one, three times a day for 3 days):
  - Take Aconite 30c for sudden attacks of panic and fear that are accompanied by restlessness and heat
  - Arsen. Alb. 30c for anxiety with restlessness, when you are worse at night, there is a thirst for cold water and a sense of dependency on other people
  - Pulsatilla 30c if you feel clingy, tearful and vulnerable

Bleeding

What is it?: Spotting or blood flow, where the blood is bright red.

What causes it?: It can be due to the sudden growth of the uterus, causing the placenta to bleed at the site of separation. If bleeding is severe, it can be an indication that miscarriage may occur (there is a 30–40 per cent risk of foetal loss during early pregnancy) and can indicate the loss of a twin in a multiple pregnancy. It can also occur as a result of a vaginal polyp or cyst suddenly becoming vascular during pregnancy, due to increased blood volume.

Important note:
• All vaginal bleeding in pregnancy needs to be investigated medically. See your doctor *immediately*. You will be sent for an ultrasound scan to see if all is well with your baby, to check if the placenta is implanted in the best possible place and to rule out ectopic pregnancy.

How can it be alleviated?:
• Rest: Once you have had a medical check-up to confirm the pregnancy is safe and continuing, take lots of rest.

Once you have consulted your GP or a hospital doctor, you may choose the following homoeopathic remedies to alleviate emotions of anxiety and fear.

• Homoeopathic remedy:
  • Aconite 30c for overwhelming fear – take one immediately and then every 6 hours for several days.
  • Phosphorus 6c every 30 minutes until you are assessed by a medical person. It helps to stop the bleeding.
  • Arnica 30c if the bleeding has been preceded by an injury, such as a fall. Take for 30 minutes for 2–3 hours.

Breathlessness
What is it?: A feeling of breathlessness that exceeds the level of cardio-vascular activity, for example, when speaking or standing.
What causes it?: The mother's cardiac output increases suddenly and the cardio-vascular system hasn't had time to catch up.

How can it be alleviated?:

- Rest as often as you can. Your heart is under an increased load at the moment, so do what you can to help it.
- A Creative Healing heart treatment is invaluable and I have known it to help immediately. See a Creative healer for this treatment.
- Homoeopathic remedy:
  - Arsen. Alb. 30c for breathlessness with anxiety, which may be worse at night in bed. Take as a single dose

Constipation

What is it?: No urge to empty the bowels and sometimes having difficulty in passing stools, leading to retention of faeces for more than 2 days in mild cases to several days in severe cases.

What causes it?: A primary cause can be the 'progesterone effect', which slows everything down. It can also be compounded by nausea, causing the mother to eat less. Ironically, it is often green leafy vegetables and other fibrous foods that are the worst culprits for inducing nausea in the early weeks, so the mother eats even less roughage. Also, some mothers tend to slow down their physical activity when they discover they are pregnant.

How can it be alleviated?:

- If you can manage it, liquidize vegetables into soups or smoothies. Try to incorporate celery, squash, broccoli, carrots, parsnips or runner beans.
- Otherwise, eat more fruit like apples, pears and berries. Do not eat bananas.
- When you need to pass stools, push as gently and slowly as you can.
- Go for short, gentle walks or try swimming once a week.
- Reflexology – ask the therapist to place emphasis on the colon reflex. (N.B. Light reflexology in the first trimester, avoiding the uterine area.)
- Ask your partner to gently perform the Creative Healing treatment on the sacrum (on the dimple area) (see page 62).
- There are several yoga poses that can help – the Child pose can help open the bowels; the Folded Lotus is an easy pose for early pregnancy before your bump gets in the way; the Rock pose can also help ease indigestion. (These

poses can be seen on the Jeyarani Yoga DVD.)

- Avoid constipation by aiding digestion. Digestive enzymes can help and are safe in pregnancy if you do not exceed one or two capsules a day. I recommend Dr Udo's or the Biocare brand of digestive enzymes.
- Probiotics help maintain gut balance – choose from the Solgar or Biocare range of probiotics. I'm not keen on bio-yogurts as we can't be sure of their shelf life and a lot of them contain added sugar.
- Homoeopathic remedies:
  - If you seem to have lost the power to defecate, with great straining even for soft stool, and if you pass hard marble-like masses, use Aluminium metallicum 6c once a day for 3 days
  - If you have a feeling of incomplete emptying of your bowels take Nux vom.6c once a day for three days
  - For a bashful stool, i.e. one that recedes when partly expelled, take Silicea 6c once a day for 3 days

Cystitis

What is it?: Infection of the urethra from the perineum. Symptoms include lower abdominal pain, urgency and increased frequency of urination. There may also be blood in the urine.

What causes it?: The female urethra is very short and therefore easily vulnerable to infection from the anus, which is in close proximity.

How can it be alleviated?:

- To prevent it, always wipe from front to back when going to the loo.
- Drink plenty of fluids. Although this means you will pass more water – which is initially painful – the fluid will be far more diluted and so less likely to give a burning sensation when you do pee. It also means you are likely to neutralize and flush out the infection faster.
- Cranberry juice is good but only drink one glass a day.
- Avoid citrus juices and caffeine.
- If symptoms continue for 3 days or there is blood in the urine, see your GP as if left untreated, the infection can travel up to your kidneys.

- Creative Healing: Heat can be taken off the abdomen using the cooling breeze, abdominal toning, pelvic drainage, the female treatment and a kidney treatment. While a few of these procedures can be done at home (see pages 53–71), you will need to visit a Creative healer to benefit from all of them.
- Reflexology: Concentrate on kidney and bladder reflexes. (N.B. Light reflexology only in the first trimester, avoiding the uterine area.)
- Homoeopathic remedies:
  - Staphisagria 30c, twice a day for 3 days, if you feel pain along the urethra and this pain eases when you pass urine
  - Cantharis 30c, twice a day for 3 days, if you have a lot of frequency, urgency and burning pain before, during and after urination

Depression

What is it?: Feeling unhappy and resentful about your pregnancy (even if the pregnancy was planned) or about your life in general.

What causes it?: Apart from the hormones of pregnancy, the demands of looking at changing your lifestyle can sometimes be overwhelming and cause depression.

How can it be alleviated?:
- A counselling session will help you get some guidelines as to how to come to terms with your pregnancy and the changes that it will bring to your life.
- Reflexology can be a mood elevator and give you a boost of energy. This will give you the impetus to exercise. (N.B. Light reflexology only in the first trimester, avoiding the uterine area.)
- Exercise will release your own endorphins, the body's mood elevators.
- Homoeopathic remedies:
  - Sepia 30c, one a day for 3 days, if you feel highly contrary with a senseless anger (you may also experience aversion to your partner)
  - Nat. Mur. 30c, once a day for 3 days, if you feel depressed associated with anger and you want to be left alone
  - Pulsatilla 30c, one a day for 3 days, if depression is associated with feeling weepy and clingy

Dizziness

What is it?: Feeling light-headed, faint, or unsteady in a standing or sitting position.

What causes it?: In early pregnancy, this can often be due to low blood pressure – although your blood volume increases in pregnancy, your blood pressure does not. Other reasons include dehydration, tiredness due to vomiting, raised blood pressure or hypoglycaemic attacks.

How can it be alleviated?:
- Sip water continuously throughout the day.
- Rest a lot.
- Stand up slowly.
- Reflexology: This helps to balance your autonomic nervous system. (N.B. Light reflexology only in the first trimester, avoiding the uterine area.)
- Homoeopathic remedies: As this is a very general complaint you will need to see a homoeopath, who will take a thorough history before providing a prescription.

Ectopic Pregnancy

What is it?: A condition where a fertilized egg is implanted outside of the uterus, such as on the fallopian tubes or on the ovaries. An ectopic pregnancy is non-viable and can endanger the mother's life.

What causes it?: Due to slow transmission of the embryo from the fallopian tube into the uterus the embryo may get implanted in the tube. This can be due to tubal adhesions or inflammation of the fallopian tube.

Important note:
- Clinical care only: See your GP *immediately*.

What can you do?:
- Take the Bach flower remedy Star of Bethlehem or Rescue Remedy – 4 drops of either in a glass of water can reduce pain and shock.
- Homoeopathic remedies:

- Aconite 30c as a single dose for shock – repeat every hour while waiting for surgery

Fatigue

What is it?: A level of tiredness that is not in keeping with your activity level; a feeling of being unable to keep up with your daily life.

What causes it?: Your cardio-vascular system is being put under pressure as your major organs grow bigger (hypertrophy) to accommodate your growing baby and the task of giving birth. Anaemia can also cause fatigue (see page 224).

How can it be alleviated?:

- If at all possible, either give up work or rearrange your hours so that you have a shorter day – i.e. go in one hour later and leave one hour earlier.
- Take a lunch break.
- Avoid travelling in the rush hour.
- Drink more water – dehydration is a major cause of tiredness. Also, your increasing blood volume requires a greater water intake.
- Don't skip meals.
- Take Bach flower remedies – Rescue Remedy, Walnut for change, and Chestnut bud to help you learn a new way of being.
- Burn peppermint oil in a diffuser for a gentle pick-me-up. It's subtle enough for you to burn on your desk at work if necessary.
- Reflexology: You can have some light reflexology if you specifically tell your therapist to avoid the pelvic and uterine areas, and the pituitary gland. Instead, he or she should work on the upper areas of the foot, concentrating on the lymphatics and gently working on the ovaries – this can boost progesterone production and help support early placenta development and implantation.
- Do your own light reflexology massage on your hands, working on lymphatic drainage. This is done by moving your fingers up and down the web-like spaces between the small bones of the palms, massaging deeply.
- You don't always have to fight the feeling. In the evenings, turn your tiredness into relaxation and have an indulgent soak in a lavender bath (up to 10

drops) before going to bed.
- Homoeopathic remedies: Due to the wide number of causes of fatigue it is best to consult a homoeopathic practitioner. However, if you tremble and shake with fatigue then Kali. Phos. 6c four times a day is recommended.
- Follow the Homoeopathic Tissue Salt Programme on pages 12–15.

Forgetfulness

What is it?: Finding it difficult to recall names, dates, conversations, where you put the keys; forgetting to lock the front door etc.

What causes it?: Oestrogen has an incredibly fluid-retentive quality that has a two-fold effect on the brain, creating a greater distance between the synapses (messaging fibres) and causing compression of the actual brain substance.

How can it be alleviated?:
- Take Rescue Remedy, one of the Bach flower remedies.
- Get into the habit of writing notes and lists.
- Reflexology is good for improving your mental acuity. (N.B. Light reflexology only in the first trimester, avoiding the uterine area.)

Heartburn

What is it?: Gastric secretions travelling back up the oesophagus from the stomach.

What causes it?: This is due to increased levels of progesterone circulating around the body and causing the sphincter muscle to overly relax. This allows tiny drops of acid to escape from the stomach and travel back up the oesophagus.

How can it be alleviated?:
- Take lots of sips of still water throughout the day (up to 3 litres) to constantly wash the lining of the oesophagus and stomach, and to dilute the acid. The water should be room temperature or, ideally, slightly warm.
- Take light exercise, such as walking, to stimulate motility of the gastro-intestinal tract.

- Reflexology: Ask your practitioner to concentrate on the oesophagus and gastro-oesophagal junction and to strictly avoid the uterine and pelvic areas.
- Apply 4 drops of lavender oil to the sternum and sweep in a downward direction.
- Avoid fizzy drinks and products such as Lucozade and glucose tablets, and anything with cane sugar.
- Add another pillow to your bed, to help prop yourself up. Avoid lying flat.
- Homoeopathic remedies:
  - For cramping indigestion with sour belches, Nux vom. 30c, one dose a day for 3 days
  - When it is worse at night and there is a metallic taste in the mouth, Merc. sol. 30c, one dose a day for 3 days
  - When it is accompanied by a desire for salt, great thirst for water and burning eructations, Nat. Mur. 30c, one dose a day for three days

Nausea (also see Vomiting, page 237)

What is it?: Often a heightened sense of smell and sensitivity to food aromas. You may not actually vomit but suffer retching and nausea. Travel sickness is often exacerbated.

What causes it?: Increased hormone levels overload the liver, meaning it cannot cleanse as quickly as it should. This is compounded by the 'progesterone effect', whereby progesterone relaxes all the smooth muscles in the body, including the oesophagus and oesophageal-gastric sphincter. Because these muscles are flaccid, it is easier for the gastric acid to pop back up into the oesophagus and cause nausea.

How can it be alleviated?:

- Sip ginger tea: Boil a root of finely sliced ginger in 1 litre (1¾ pints) water for 20 minutes. Strain and serve first thing in the morning. If you want to sweeten it, allow it to cool and add one teaspoon of honey (it is important that the tea is cooled first as honey becomes toxic when warmed).
- Sip room-temperature water, constantly. Do not gulp.
- Eliminate caffeine from your diet.

- Cut out wheat – this will make an immediate difference.
- Creative Healing is good for a digestive tune-up. Have the General Treatment (pages 55–64), Back and spine treatment (pages 64–7) and Abdominal toning (pages 67–8). Emphasis should be clearing the lymphatics. See a Creative Healer for a full treatment which should include pancreatic and liver drainage, and finished off with a heart treatment.
- Light reflexology can be effective – again ask your therapist to keep away from the pelvic and uterine area, and to concentrate on the stomach, oesophagus, kidneys and liver. The therapist's intention should be to detoxify and drain.
- Drink peppermint tea (do not have this if you are taking homoeopathic remedies). If you wish to make your own, you'll find a recipe on page 301.
- There are sometimes psychological factors at the root of nausea and vomiting, and these can be addressed through hypnotherapy. This is more often the case with older mothers who feel fearful, at some level, about the huge mental shift of giving up their current lifestyle for a new one.
- Travel sickness bands can abate nausea in pregnancy too. They work by applying pressure to the Nei Kuan point in the wrist.
- Finally, there are instances when nothing seems to help, except bland food like buttered toast. This is fine for getting you through the worst of these early weeks, but it is very important that you do not put on extra weight at this point in the pregnancy as it will be difficult to shift later on and can lead mothers to feel depressed.
- Homoeopathic remedies: (For all the remedies below, the dose is one, three times a day, for 3 days.)
  - Sepia 30c, the classic remedy for morning sickness, is suited if you feel sick at the sight, smell and even the thought of food. You might also feel nauseous all the time
  - Ipecac. 30c if you feel nauseated all the time
  - Nux vom. 30c if your tummy feels bloated and tender with marked flatulence and you crave chocolate or something sweet
  - Nat. Mur. 30c if you have nausea accompanied with a craving for salt and a thirst for water

- Arsenicum 30c for persistent nausea and vomiting that leads to exhaustion. This remedy is for you if you feel well with hot drinks but don't like cold drinks
- Pulsatilla 30c if you get more nauseated when eating fatty foods and if you hate hot environments and feel weepy

Pelvic Pain

What is it?: In pregnancy pelvic pain is situated in the lower abdomen and around the bladder and base of the uterus.

What causes it?: In the sixth week of pregnancy there is a sudden growth of the uterus, which stretches the uterine ligaments and pulls on the peritoneum – the lining of the inner wall of the abdominal cavity. This pain can be referred into the pelvic area. Pain can also be caused by inflammation and stress on the joints within the pelvis.

How can it be alleviated?:
- Cranio-sacral therapy can give you fascial release.
- Reflexology will decongest muscles and tendons by improving lymphatic drainage. Work thoroughly around the pelvic reflexes situated around the ankles, avoiding the uterine area.
- Bowen therapy is an extremely efficient technique for pelvic pain. Ask the therapist for full core-level moves with pelvic release techniques.
- A Creative Healing General Treatment (pages 55–64) together with a Back and spine treatment (pages 64–7) will help.
- Homoeopathic remedies: (For all the remedies below, the dose is one, three times a day, for 3 days.)
  - Arnica 30c if joints feel painful and sensitive to touch
  - Ruta grav. 30c if there is a sense of weakness made worse by over-exertion and when the pain improves on lying down and with warmth

Thrush

What is it?: Overgrowth of the fungus Candida Albicans, which normally occurs in the vagina. It causes severe vulval irritation and a curdy, white discharge.

What causes it?: Candida is a normal inhabitant of the gut, however, if there is a predominance of carbohydrates in your diet, there is an overgrowth of Candida in the gut that then spills over into the adjacent vagina. In the non-pregnant woman, the vaginal pH is acidic and Candida cannot survive in this acidic medium. However, in pregnancy the vaginal secretions are alkaline and Candida flourishes in this environment.

How can it be alleviated?:

- It is very important to seriously reduce your intake of refined sugar and even cut down on general carbohydrate intake. Eating lots of green leafy vegetables will help to balance your gut flora.
- Probiotics: I recommend the Biocare range or Solgar brand. Pre-mixed liquid drinks of probiotics or yoghurts must be sugar-free and well inside their sell-by date.
- Drink a glass of water to which you have added 1 teaspoon of apple cider vinegar and 1 teaspoon dark unblended (i.e. from one source) honey.
- Mix one drop of tea tree essential oil (Melaleuca alternifolia) in 5ml of virgin olive oil, then dip an index finger in this mixture and swish it around within your vagina twice a day for two or three days. It works a dream!
- Homoeopathic remedies:
  - Candida Albicans 30c, once a day for 4 or 5 days

Urinary Retention

What is it?: Acute retention of urine. It is extremely painful and usually occurs before 16 weeks.

What causes it?: An acutely retroverted uterus (the top of the uterus has folded back towards the rectum) that has impacted into the pelvic space, putting pressure on the neck of the bladder.

How can it be alleviated:

- Try an ice-pack initially on your perineum.
- If the above doesn't work and you are in a great deal of pain, you may need to be catheterized hence you need to go to your nearest A & E department.

Vomiting

What is it?: 'Morning sickness' is a misnomer – you can be sick any time of day, although many people do suffer most in the morning, when their hormone levels surge. There is also an increased level of nausea and vomiting in multiple pregnancies, because your body is producing twice as many hormones, so excessive sickness is often an indication you might be carrying twins or triplets.

What causes it?: Basically, hormones. Increased oestrogen levels and human chorionic gonadotrophin (HCG) can upset the emetic centre of the brain – this area of the brain 'polices' acceptable levels of circulating nutrients and hormones. For example, if you eat something unusual the brain may interpret it as a poison and command the body to vomit in response. The emetic centre has been proven to be sensitive to high levels of oestrogen. It is a well-known fact that vomiting is a common side-effect of the contraceptive pill (which creates a pseudo-pregnancy state) because it introduces marginally higher-than-normal levels of oestrogen to the body to inhibit ovulation. Nausea and vomiting eventually subside between 12–16 weeks, as the mother's emetic centre slowly readjusts to the higher levels of pregnancy hormones in circulation.

How can it be alleviated?:
- For helpful methods see the Nausea entry on page 233.

Important note – exceptions to the rule:
- Abnormal vomiting can be a symptom of a molar pregnancy, which occurs when there is a chromosomal abnormality in the male chromosome. This means that the uterus doesn't develop a foetus but rather the placenta undergoes a hydrophic degeneration, where every little end vessel of the placenta forms a vesicle, resembling a bunch of grapes. The uterus is typically larger than expected for gestation. Other symptoms include bleeding and blood tests reveal extraordinarily high levels of the hormone human chorionic gonadotrophin (HCG). You must see your GP if you are suffering from excessive sickness.
- Hyperemesis Gravidaerum is a severe form of vomiting in pregnancy, causing weight loss and leading to fluid and electrolyte imbalance. The dehydration must be clinically corrected and hospitalization is usually required. See your GP.

Clinical Notes: Vomiting and gagging throughout pregnancy

Belinda, 42 years old, first pregnancy

Belinda presented at 30 weeks' gestation. Severe vomiting (hyperemesis) due to abnormally increased saliva secretion (sialation) in pregnancy meant she had lost three stone in weight during her pregnancy and she looked deficient in nutrients.

I gave her some Creative Healing sessions, concentrating on the heart and hiatus hernia treatments, and liver and pancreatic treatments. During the sessions, I also talked her through a self-hypnosis visualization to sedate the nervous system and remove any fear that might be underlying the symptoms. Within three weeks, these techniques had helped reduce salivation to acceptable levels.

Due to the powerful effects of the treatments, she felt emotionally strong and physically well prepared enough for a home birth. She asked me to attend her birth to give her birth support and she proceeded to have a wonderful labour and water birth with no drugs, minimal pushing and an intact perineum.

The Second Trimester

Your Body in the Second Trimester

The greatest thing about the second trimester is the fact that your chance of miscarriage now drops dramatically. Your uterus has risen above your pelvic bones now and by the time you exit this stage, it will be up at your rib cage. You will also have a dark pigmented line, called the linea nigra running down the centre of your tummy – this is due to high hormone levels and will disappear after the birth. For the same reason your nipples are darker too, your hair is thicker and your nails stronger. It is during this trimester that you will move out of your normal clothes and into pregnancy-wear. You probably haven't slept on your tummy for a good few weeks now but you'll probably also find it uncomfortable to sleep on your back after 20 weeks. As your bump rapidly swells, this is when you risk developing stretch marks. They tend to be hereditary (if your mother had them, you're likely to) but you can better your chances of minimizing them by keeping the skin moisturized and supple. Best of all though, this is the period in which you hit the all-important halfway mark. You can then start counting down to meeting your baby.

Your Baby in the Second Trimester

Your baby begins to take on a more human appearance during this trimester, with its head – which was previously half its length – now being overtaken by the body's growth. Your baby will also become more active now. From 16 weeks (or before if this isn't your first pregnancy), you will feel the first kicks and rolls and there will be lots and lots of them – this is the period of greatest activity as the baby has plenty of room to move around.

The baby also begins to distinguish and recognize your voice, and to react to light too. Its reflexes are also maturing – if its fingers inadvertently touch the soles of its feet, the toes curl down, and it can suck its thumb. Your baby is now covered in vernix caseosa, a white substance that protects the baby's skin during its long immersion in the amniotic fluids, and, at 26 weeks, its body becomes covered in a super-soft downy hair called lanugo.

Most exciting of all, however, is that after 24 weeks, your baby is considered 'viable', as it has an 85 per cent chance of survival if it is born at this stage. Three weeks later, your baby opens its eyes for the first time and takes little breaths (although it's water, not air that your baby is breathing).

Trimester Two: A–Z Guide

Back Pain (also see Back Pain in the Third Trimester, page 254)
What is it?: Pain that originates at any point along the whole of the back, from the base of your skull to the tip of your tail bone.
What causes it?: Common causes are bad posture and shifting weight distribution due to your baby growing rather rapidly in your abdominal cavity. This results in an exaggerated lumbar curvature that is called a lumbar lordosis. The

resultant pull on all your back muscles and nerves can cause acute or chronic back pain. Laxity in the spinal ligaments, due to the 'progesterone effect', can also contribute to lumbar lordosis.

How can it be alleviated?:
- Creative Healing: The Back and spine treatment (pages 64–7) can effectively loosen the back muscles, while the re-positioning techniques correct poor alignment of the vertebrae. This treatment applies all of the principles of Creative Healing. You can visit a Creative healer for it.
- Homoeopathic remedies (for all, take one dose, three times a day for three days):
  - Bellis perennis 30c is for you if you suffer with backache associated with general muscle aches, especially in the legs, and walking is difficult
  - Kali. Carb. 30c if your back pain is mostly in the small of your back, radiating to the hips, and gets worse in cold weather
  - Nat. mur. 30c if you have mostly low back pain that is relieved by firm pressure and support in the small of the back
  - Rhus tox. 30c if your back pain is worse when you begin to move but improves after you have been moving around a bit – and if warmth makes it feel better
  - The Homoeopathic Tissue Salt Programme can act as a prophylaxis against back pain (see pages 12–13)

Fibroid Uterus
What is it?: Fibroids are spherical muscle overgrowths on the surface, muscle wall or inner lining of the uterus. They can cause abdominal pain.
What causes it?: The fibroids grow rapidly in response to oestrogen, an important hormone of pregnancy that is synthesized in large amounts by the placenta. Pain results when the rapid growth of the fibroids outstrips its blood supply, causing the centre of the fibroid to undergo necrosis (cell death and tissue liquefaction). Sometimes the fibroids may grow so large that, if they're in the lower uterine area, they may obstruct the delivery of the baby, necessitating a caesarean. A very large fibroid uterus that becomes painful can precipitate miscarriage, or premature labour.

How can it be alleviated?:

- The only way is to seek to calm down the uterine response to oestrogens. I have used visualization techniques to cool down the fibroids and visualize them shrinking comfortably. Along with this I have also applied Creative Healing in the specific combination below, which has been very effective.
- Creative Healing: The techniques of cupping to take heat off the uterus (see page 54) and abdominal toning (see page 67–8) and pelvic drainage (see page 68–9) have slowed down the proliferation of the fibroids and reduced inflammation. This has then restored comfort within the abdominal cavity. I recommend lavender essential oil (10 drops in a teaspoon of virgin olive oil) to perform these techniques. These treatments should ideally be done on a daily basis.
- Reflexology: A general all-round treatment can be very effective in calming you down and helping redistribution of energy throughout your body so that the uterus can relax and heal.
- Rest plays an important part in calming down inflammation within the uterus.
- Homoeopathic remedies:
  - You could take one dose of Arnica 30c to ease the pain
  - Following this, see a homoeopath

Headaches/Migraines

What is it?: Pulsing or consistent pain behind the eyes and across the head.

What causes it?: Headaches in pregnancy can originate from muscle tension in the neck, due to postural changes and stress, or eyestrain. They can also be exacerbated by hormonal changes, which can lead to vasodilatation in the small blood vessels in the brain. Blocked sinuses can mimic migraines.

Important note: Severe persistent headaches need medical investigation – if you experience these you should see your GP.

How can they be alleviated?:

- Drink plenty of water.
- If you are reading from a screen or book for long periods of time, break away

every 15 minutes and let your gaze rest on a spot in the middle distance for two minutes. This relaxes your eye muscles.

- If the pain is mild, go for a short walk. Fresh air and gentle cardio-vascular activity can really help to 'blow away the cobwebs'.
- Eliminate the following foods from your diet:
  - Wheat – it is proven to cause fluid retention and can cause slight swelling in the neck muscles, leading to tension and headaches.
  - Cheese, chocolate, red meats, red wine and red kidney beans. This is because they contain a high content of tyramine, which is a trigger for headaches or migraines.
- Creative Healing: The treatments for headaches and migraines are very effective in helping this condition – they include treating the neck and the sinuses. See a Creative healer.
- Reflexology has been known to be beneficial. Emphasis should be on the brain, head and neck, sinus and stomach areas.
- Homoeopathic remedies: see a homoeopath, as there are many suitable remedies and you need to be evaluated carefully.

Herpes Gestationis

What is it?: Blistering skin eruptions, usually occurring in the second and third trimesters.

What causes it?: This is a rare disease, not a virus. It can occur when your immune system is challenged by the stresses and strains of pregnancy. It usually presents as urticarial spots (like raised wheals), which then blister.

How can it be alleviated?:
- Homoeopathic remedies:
  - Nat. Mur. 6c three times a day for three days, if there is a desire for salt, a thirst for water, and/or depressed mood
  - Rhus tox. 6c three times a day for three days, if there is restlessness

Herpes Simplex

What is it?: Herpes Simplex Type 1 presents as ulcers and sores on the mouth and nose; Simplex Type 2 occurs in the genital area – the vulva, vagina, labia and cervix.

What causes it?: Herpes during pregnancy indicates a lowered immune status.

How can it be alleviated?:
- Boost your diet with oily fish and leafy green vegetables.
- Homoeopathic remedies:
  - Alternate Nat. Mur. 6c three times a day for three days with Rhus tox. 6c three times a day for three days
  - The Homoeopathic Tissue Salt Programme (see pages 12–13) may offer prophylaxis against this

Hip Pain

What is it?: Sharp or achy pains in the hip and pelvic areas.

What causes it?: It is associated with stretching ligaments in the pelvic area as your uterus grows and your pelvis expands due to progesterone. But excess mobility of these joints can be painful. You may be surprised to learn that there are fascial connections between the jaw and the hip joints and tension in the jaw area can affect the hip joints. Before man evolved to become upright, we were on all-fours and the jaw hung forward, parallel to the ground. However, walking upright places a great strain on the cranial base and the jaw joint (temporo-mandibular joint). Releasing this area greatly increases the mobility of the pelvis as a whole and helps the baby's head to engage and be born easily.

How can it be alleviated?:
- Bowen therapy helps your muscles to readjust and compensate for the extra load that you carry within your womb and abdomen. Ask your practitioner to treat the temporo-mandibular joint (T-M joint).
- Creative Healing: the General Treatment (pages 55–64) and the Back and spine treatment (pages 64–7) can help, especially if given in combination with the Bowen technique. See a Creative healer who ideally also knows

Bowen techniques.
- Homoeopathic remedy: (take one dose, twice a day, for 3 days)
  - Rhus tox. 30c if you feel worse after exertion and worse in the morning
  - Hip and groin pain benefits from Bellis perennis 30c

Immunological Stress (frequent illnesses)

What is it?: Persistent and recurring coughs and colds.

What causes it?: It can be caused by nutritional/vitamin/mineral deficiencies as the baby takes what it needs from the mother's body for growth and development, thereby depleting her supply. It can also point to emotional stress and feeling 'run down' due to the demands of daily life.

How can it be alleviated?:
- Supplements: take pre-natal vitamins and minerals along with probiotics and digestive enzymes. (For stockists, see Appendix C, pages 311–12.)
- Diet:
  - Eat whole grains with steamed vegetables and sprouting seeds i.e. alfalfa, mung beans
  - Soak 6 almonds in a glass of water overnight and in the morning peel off the skins and eat them one by one, chewing well. These contain amazingly nourishing enzymes
  - Add cinnamon, thyme, oregano, peppercorns and bay leaves to your soups and foods as they are immuno-stimulants
- Bach Flower Remedies: Take Rescue Remedy and the Remedy Olive for exhaustion. Place 4 drops of each in a glass of water and sip slowly throughout the day.
- Creative Healing: To tone up the pancreas, liver and spleen – see a Creative healer.
- Reflexology: Have a treatment once a week, emphasizing the thyroid, pituitary, adrenals, liver, spleen and the gut area to stimulate immune function.
- Try a massage with immuno-stimulatory essential oils – there are many but try the easily available ones such as neroli (orange blossom), which is excellent, tea tree (Melaleuca alternifolia), eucalyptus globus, lavender (Latifolia),

rose, sandalwood, thyme (Thymus vulgaris – linaloliferum), vetiver and frankincense. As a general rule use 4 drops of 1 or 2 of the above oils in a teaspoon of virgin olive oil and use for massage, using circular movements on your back and downwards along your limbs.

- Homoeopathic remedies:
  - The Homoeopathic Tissue Salt Programme (see pages 12–13)
  - Your constitution will need to be taken into account before a specific remedy is recommended, so see a homoeopath

Insomnia

What is it?: An inability to initiate or maintain natural sleep.

What causes it?: Common factors include emotional stress (such as moving house, work worries, relationship issues). Later in pregnancy, it can be caused by positional problems as the heavier uterus makes sleeping in certain positions uncomfortable or impossible.

How can it be alleviated?:

- Drink warm milk (goat's milk or rice milk) before going to bed – this acts as a sedative and induces sleepiness.
- Bach Flower Remedies: Rescue Remedy – 4 drops in a glass of water 3 times a day. Sip slowly.
- Half an hour before going to bed, have a warm (not hot) bath containing 10 drops of lavender essential oil and/or basil.
- If you are still awake 20 minutes after going to bed, get up and practise your yoga routine.
- Sleep with the window open. By cooling your body temperature a little, you mimic the natural lower base temperature the body adopts in sleep.
- Cranio-sacral treatments have been known to help with insomnia by restoring cranial rhythms.
- Homoeopathic remedies: This merits a visit to the homoeopath as there are a variety of suitable remedies and the homoeopath will help you to hone in on the right one for you.

Jaundice:

What is it?: A yellowing of the skin and the whites of the eyes.

What causes it?: It can happen at any stage and can be due to cholestasis or a small gall stone blocking your bile duct – this can be very painful. Rarely, a viral infection of the liver can cause jaundice.

How can it be alleviated?:

- Clinical care only – no self-medication. Visit your GP for a blood test and other investigations. Alternatively, visit an Ayurvedic practitioner. Ayurvedic physicians are extremely effective in treating jaundice – this is well-documented in India.
- Homoeopathic remedies: See a homoeopath.

Leg Cramps

What is it?: Sudden and painful shortening of the calf and hamstring muscles in the legs.

What causes it?: Most often attributed to nutritional and mineral deficiencies, such as iron, magnesium, calcium or salt insufficiency.

How can it be alleviated?:

- To prevent leg cramps, ensure you take pre-natal vitamin and mineral supplements (see pages 11–12).
- Homoeopathic remedies:
  - Calc. Carb. 30c, take one twice a day for 3 days if symptoms are worse at night in bed
  - Sepia 30c, one twice a day for 3 days, for the general cramps of pregnancy
  - The Homoeopathic Tissue Salt Programme for prophylaxis (see pages 12–13)

Low-lying Placenta

What is it?: When the edge of the placenta is implanted close to the inner opening of the cervix.

What causes it?: The placenta can implant on the anterior, posterior or lateral walls of the uterus – it is entirely random.

How can it be alleviated?:
- As the uterus grows with the baby during pregnancy, the placenta is naturally stretched up and away from the cervical opening.
- If it doesn't grow away, the term given is Placenta Praevia – see separate entry in the third trimester.

Nose Bleeds
What is it?: Sudden, unexplained bleeding from the nose.

What causes it?: In pregnancy they are often the result of the 'progesterone effect' (progesterone causes thickening and proliferation of mucous membranes). The nasal mucosa can become very congested and eventually break down. Hay fever, sinusitis and nasal polyps can also cause nose bleeds, as does raised blood pressure. All nose bleeds should be investigated to rule out high blood pressure.

How can it be alleviated?:
- When the nose bleed occurs, throw your head back so that your nose is high up in the air as this can slow down the bleeding. Pinch the bridge of your nose firmly for at least 5 minutes, then apply an ice compress to your nose.
- Creative Healing: See a Creative healer to treat your adenoids and sinuses.
- Homoeopathic remedies:
  - Phosphorus 30c, one a day for 3 days, if you are depressed, irritable and restless in bed
  - Ferr. met. 30c, one a day for 3 days, if you are feeling anxious about your health and sensitive

Obstetric Cholestasis
What is it?: Excessive itching of the skin all over the body but without a rash. It usually occurs in mid-trimester.

What causes it?: It is a rare condition associated with pregnancy. It is thought that oestrogen produced by the placenta causes dilatation of the bile ducts, which slows down the movement of bile flow in the liver. This leads to a build up of bile salts (bilirubin) in the blood and high levels of circulating bile salts causes itching of the skin. Liver function tests can indicate the severity of the condition.

If the condition persists, obstetricians generally advise early delivery of the baby (by 37 weeks of pregnancy) as there is a reported risk of stillbirths in those who have rising levels of bile salts in circulation as they go towards term.

Important note:
• Visit your GP if you suspect you may have this. You will be given liver function tests and a scan, checking your liver for evidence of bile duct dilatation and gallstones.

How can it be alleviated?:
• Vitamin K will be given to you orally to help blood clotting (it will also be given to your baby after birth).
• Diet:
  • Go on a low-fat mostly vegetarian diet
  • Give up wheat – choose rice, millet and buckwheat instead
  • Minimize intake of dairy products
  • It goes without saying, but give up alcohol
• Creative Healing: See a Creative healer for a liver treatment.
• Reflexology: Have a general treatment with an emphasis on liver drainage.
• Ayurveda offers excellent remedies – consult an Ayurvedic physician.
• Homoeopathic remedies: a homoeopath can help to ease the condition.

Pruritis (Itching)
What is it?: Generalized itching (all over the body). If there is generalized itching it is important to have a liver function test to rule out Obstetric Cholestasis (see above).
What causes it?: Causes could include dilation of the skin capillaries (possibly due to the 'progesterone effect'); dry skin; environmental pollutants; (see above for itching associated with Cholestasis).
How can it be alleviated?:
• Moisturize your skin to keep it supple and elastic as it stretches.

- Hydrated skin is more elastic, so drink lots of water.
  - Pulsatilla 30c can be given, one dose twice a day for 3 days

Thankfully, there is usually total remission after delivery.

Restless Legs Syndrome (see also Restless legs in the Third Trimester, pages 269–70)

What is it?: An involuntary twitching of the legs, which makes it difficult for the mother to sit or lie still. Some mothers describe it as a feeling of 'electricity' running inside the legs. This tends to happen in particular at night, when the involuntary movements can disturb or prevent sleep.

What causes it?: The cause is uncertain, but can be associated with general fluid retention that swells up the covering of nerves (nerve sheaths) during pregnancy. Vitamin and mineral deficiencies can contribute to the irritability of the peripheral nerves. Old spinal injuries may manifest in this way.

How can it be alleviated?:

- Place your legs in a half-filled bath of cool water, to numb the sensation.
- Ayurvedic treatment offers hot oil massages, oil pouring (Pirichal) and compresses that can feed and soothe the nervous system.
- Homoeopathic remedies:
  - Rhus tox. 30c, one dose twice a day for 3 days, if you like a warm bed and hot drinks.
  - Zinc 30c, one dose twice a day for 3 days, if you feel depressed and irritable
  - Use the Homoeopathic Tissue Salt Programme (see pages 12–13) as a prophylaxis

Sacro-iliac Pain

What is it?: Severe shooting pains over the sacrum, going down into the hip and buttock areas.

What causes it?: Caused by laxity of the sacro-iliac ligaments due to the 'progesterone effect'. Can also be caused by old injuries manifesting themselves.

How can it be alleviated?:

- A support belt can be helpful.

- Bouncing on your toes in a squatting position for a minute at a time can reposition the joints.
- Bowen treatment: All core moves should be included in the treatment with emphasis on the hip and pelvis.
- Cranio-sacral treatment: The therapist should treat the focal points and fascial unwinding.
- Creative Healing: General Treatment (pages 55–64) and Back and spine treatment (see pages 64–7). In severe cases see a Creative Healer.
- Reflexology: Emphasis in the treatment should be on the sacrum, sciatic nerve areas and colon.
- Homoeopathic remedies (for all, take one dose three times a day for three days):
  - Rhus tox. 30c if you are better with movements and warm compresses
  - Ruta grav. 30c if there is an associated weakness in the joints and limping

Sciatica

What is it?: Searing pain radiating from the mid-point of the buttock, down the back of the thigh and the side of the leg, right down to the little toe.

What causes it?: Pure sciatica usually occurs when the sciatic nerve is compressed at the midpoint of the buttock, between two buttock muscles (pyriformis muscle). However, often sciatica is associated with several pelvic muscles being chronically inflamed. A multi-disciplinary approach is required to relieve muscle spasm and decongest the area.

How can it be alleviated?:

- The pain can be reduced by relaxing the buttock muscles with simple massage using muscle relaxing essential oils such as lavender (4 drops) in virgin olive oil (10ml).
- Take warm baths. You can add 10 drops of lavender essential oil and basil, which is relaxing to the central nervous system.
- Reduce anxiety and stressful situations by changing your lifestyle.
- Yoga stretching e.g spinal twists will help (do this under supervision).

- Diet: give up wheat and sugar, which causes fluid retention in muscles and nerve sheaths.
- Creative Healing: Decongesting the sacrum (pages 62–4) will help. See a Creative healer.
- Bowen: This is excellent for treating acute conditions and can give you instant muscle relaxation.
- Cranio-sacral therapy.
- Reflexology: Ask for an emphasis on lymphatic drainage, the spine, neck, sacrum and the whole digestive tract.
- Homoeopathic remedies:
  - Mag. Phos. 30c, one dose mixed with a third of a glass of water then slowly sip and stir, sip and stir (repeated stirring makes the remedy more potent)
  - Homoeopathic Tissue Salt Programme (see pages 12–13) as a prophylaxis.

The Third Trimester

Your Body in the Final Trimester

You're on the home stretch – your baby's nutritional needs reach their peak during this trimester, so be really vigilant about your diet and make sure you take plenty of protein, vitamin C, folic acid, iron and calcium. Your uterus is so high now, it's pressing up against your diaphragm and possibly leaving you breathless, so do some yoga stretches. Stretching the chest area up and away from the uterus will provide temporary relief. You'll find though that between weeks 34 and 36, your baby's head engages, so the baby moves down into your pelvis, creating more room and space at the top of the uterus. Your breasts are probably several cup sizes larger now, as your milk is stored and ready for the baby, and your back is wider too, as the baby's size pushes out your rib cage.

Your Baby in the Final Trimester

By now your baby weighs nearly 3lb and in these last few weeks, it is going to put on a lot more, roughly ½ lb a week, ready for life outside the womb. All the major organs are now fully matured and if you are having a boy, his testicles should have descended from his abdomen into his scrotum. You will find that the baby moves about less within the womb, as there is less room. Brain growth is rapid – a most wonderful thought for you to ponder on is that your baby is now dreaming.

Trimester Three: A–Z Guide

Back Pain (see also Back Pain in the Second Trimester, page 240)
What is it?: Pain that originates from any point along the whole of the back from the base of your skull to the tip of your tail bone.
What causes it?: In this last trimester, it is generally due to the greater strain on the back muscles as your baby grows heavier within your womb. Although of course, it may also be due to the reasons listed in this entry in the Second Trimester (see page 240).

How can it be alleviated?:
- Rest when you can. Lying on your side will take the baby's weight both off your back and stomach muscles.
- If your back pain is due to bad posture, have some Creative Healing. Start with the General Treatment (pages 55–64) followed by the Back and spine treatment (pages 64–7). The Back and spine treatment will effectively loosen the back muscles, while the re-positioning techniques correct poor alignment of the vertebrae. This treatment applies all of the principles of Creative Healing – visit a Creative healer.
- Homoeopathic remedies – choose an appropriate remedy from the list below (for all, take one three times a day for three days):
  - Bellis perennis 30c is for you if you suffer with backache associated with general muscle aches, especially in the legs, and walking is difficult
  - Kali. Carb. 30c if your back pain is mostly in the small of your back, radiating to the hips, and gets worse in cold weather

- Nat. Mur. 30c if you have mostly low back pain that is relieved by firm pressure
- Rhus tox. 30c if your back pain is worse when you begin to move but improves after you have been moving around a bit and if warmth makes it feel better
- The Homoeopathic Tissue Salt Programme acts as a prophylaxis against back pain (see pages 12–13)

Breech Presentation

What is it?: A breech presentation is when the foetus within the womb presents with the head at the top of the uterus and the buttocks (fully-flexed breech) or feet (footling breech) at the lower end of the uterus, close to the inner aspect of the cervix (within the amniotic sac). Normal presentation is the vertex position, when the baby's head is in line with the opening of the cervix and the vagina.

What causes it?: Up to 32 weeks of pregnancy, the baby is fairly mobile and may lie in several positions in the womb. Between weeks 32 and 36, the amount of amniotic fluid in the womb reduces as the baby grows bigger and the baby's position usually stabilizes into the vertex position. Breech presentation may occur at this time because:

- Some mothers have different uterine shapes i.e. a bicornuate (heart-shaped) uterus, which is a developmental abnormality. This allows less manoeuvrability for the baby within the womb hence the baby finds it difficult to settle into the head-down position.
- An obstruction in the lower part of the uterus, i.e. a low-lying placenta, fibroids or a pelvic ovarian tumour, prevents the baby's head from dropping down.
- Psychological causes include deep-seated maternal fear of the birth process and/or mothering.
- If the mother has a very small android (male-shaped) or narrow, cone-like pelvis there is less room for the baby to move around easily.

How can you encourage the baby to turn?:

- Moxa sticks – used in Chinese medicine – have a 76 per cent success rate in turning breech babies. Between weeks 32 and 36, your therapist or partner should daily heat the Moxa sticks and circle them, in little circles, as close as is comfortable, to the outer tip of your little toe, one at a time. This serves to heat the meridian channel that runs up to the uterus, gently warming the womb and encouraging the baby to move. Do this for a total of 10 minutes.
- Hypnotherapy and visualization: A one-to-one hypnotherapy session can release fear in both mother and baby and allow repositioning of the baby into the head-down position within the womb.
- By kneeling down on all fours with your bottom in the air and your head resting on your hands, you force the baby into the 'hammock' of your bump, encouraging it to turn. Practise every day as much as possible, for a minimum of 10 minutes at a time.
- Cranio-sacral therapy: This works on a physical and emotional level. A good therapist can also work on the baby through the mother's abdomen.
- Acupuncture.
- Homoeopathic remedies:
  - Ideally this should be supervised by a homoeopathic practitioner. Pulsatilla 30c can be taken from 36 weeks to encourage breech/transverse babies to turn. Take one twice a day for three days, stop when you feel a significant movement of your baby, then go and have a check-up with your midwife or doctor to see if the baby has turned. If the baby has not turned, stop the remedy for 2 days and then take the remedy again twice a day for 3 days.

Coccyx Pain

What is it?: Pain or numbness in the tailbone that makes sitting down deeply uncomfortable.

What causes it?: It is usually caused by a previous, unresolved trauma to the coccyx that becomes inflamed due to the greater load put on the spine by pregnancy.

How can it be alleviated?:

- Sit on a cushion whenever possible.

- Creative Healing: Decongest the sacrum and lift up the tissues on either side of the coccyx. For details of how to do this see pages 62–4.
- Bowen treatment: Full core treatment followed by moves on the sacrum, coccyx and all the pelvic moves.
- Homoeopathic remedies (for remedies below take one 3 times a day for 3 days):
  - Hypericum 30c if there are shooting pains, numbness or tingling pains associated with injury
  - Arnica 30c if the coccyx is painful to touch and feels very bruised
  - Arnica cream applied over the coccyx area can be soothing

Eclampsia

What is it?: High blood pressure associated with swellings and loss of protein in the urine. The blood pressure tends to be dangerously high and can lead to convulsions. It is quite rare to see this condition in developed countries although it is quite common in countries where there is less pre-natal monitoring. Common complications include 'small-for-dates' babies. However, it can cause convulsions, early labour, bleeding, and even death.

What causes it?: It is usually due to a poor diet that is deficient in essential nutrients. Recently it has been suggested that it may be caused by a low-grade infection in the placenta. Autoimmune causes have been suggested but not proved.

Important note: This condition is extremely serious and hospital admission is mandatory.

How can it be alleviated?:
- A homoeopath may be able to help minimize long-term damage.

Gestational Diabetes

What is it?: Abnormally raised blood-sugar levels in a pregnant mother may be associated with sugar detected in the urine on routine ante-natal checking. Mothers could have increased thirst and tiredness.

What causes it?: In gestational diabetes, the placental hormones antagonize (work against) the action of insulin and this causes high blood-sugar levels in the mother. The baby's insulin production is normal and therefore the excess blood sugars are rapidly snapped up by the baby and the baby may suddenly grow bigger than the anticipated size for gestation. The mother's pancreas does not seem to have the capacity to produce additional insulin to overcome the blocking effects of the placental hormones. It can begin around 24 weeks but is commonly observed around 28 weeks. Gestational diabetes usually disappears after the baby is born.

How can it be alleviated?:
- All mothers with gestational diabetes have to be closely monitored by their obstetrician.
- Creative Healing: I have found this invaluable in dramatically normalizing blood sugars in the mother. A pancreatic treatment generally does the trick. This is simple enough to perform at home on a weekly basis. This technique can be taught to you by a Creative healer or you can learn it by watching the Creative Healing DVD (see page 314).
- Diet:
  - Restrict your intake of carbohydrates
  - Stop eating fruit and drinking fruit juices
  - Triple your intake of vegetables (but not the carbohydrate-full ones such as potatoes)
  - Drink 2 litres (3½ pints) of water a day
- Supplements:
  - Vitamins and mineral supplements should be taken, with special emphasis on chromium, selenium and magnesium to control your cravings for sugars
  - Ambrotose supplements provide a combination of 8 essential sugars; these do not provide calories but enable cell-to-cell communication within your body and especially your brain, reducing cravings for sweet things. (For supplies see Appendix C, page 312.)

Clinical Notes: Gestational Diabetes
Diana, 35 years old, first pregnancy, family history of diabetes

Diana wanted a home birth and to keep out of hospital at all costs, due to negative hospital experiences in the past. She enrolled on the programme at 24 weeks – very stressed and still at work. She was clinically normal, however, a holistic assessment revealed that she was tense and very tight in her back. She had put on more weight than she should have at this stage of pregnancy and was puffy around her face and eyes. She looked tired and unwell.

A reflexology assessment confirmed she was holding tension in her back muscles, neck and shoulders, and even in the area of the brain reflex. (Mothers always laugh when I say that their brain is stressed out!) During the reflexology sessions, the feet were quite tight and had a toxic feel to them i.e. they sweated profusely when specific areas were deeply worked on. The feet also indicated, even during the early sessions between 24 to 28 weeks, that the pancreatic reflex area was very nodular (the pancreas is responsible for insulin production). Appropriate action was taken by applying the Creative Healing pancreatic treatment on the abdomen.

I had difficulty initially in making her understand that pregnancy is a special event and that she had to consider taking time off work. She remained rather stubborn in her opinion that she could take all the stress of work and that her methods of trying to relax at home were sufficient. However, her body gave her a powerful signal that she was overdoing things when her blood sugar levels went up and her blood pressure became slightly elevated. The hospital wanted to do further tests, suspecting early gestational diabetes, and told her that a home birth was not recommended, as the baby may need to go into an incubator after the birth.

I devised an intensive version of the programme for her to get her birthfit quickly and reduce her blood sugar levels. I advised her to cut out wheat and sugar; to restrict carbohydrates to one small cupful three times a day; to take four cupfuls of vegetables at lunch and dinner; to have two tablespoons at least of olive oil drizzled onto steamed vegetables (not microwaved as this is a toxic method of food preparation); to take antioxidants (Polbax, two tablets three times a day); to have twice weekly Creative Healing treatments; to do deep muscle relaxation techniques and to visualize the beta cells of the pancreas making more of her own insulin for her.

Within a week, Diana felt a lot better and more energetic. Her blood sugar levels and blood pressure normalized after two weeks and she was declared by her local maternity unit to be free of gestational diabetes. Much to her relief the paediatrician said she could have a home birth.

Much to my relief, by the time she was 34 weeks she decided of her own accord that she would give up work. After several weeks of one-to-one therapy she was more relaxed and ready to give birth – and her birth story surprised both of us.

She went into labour in the early hours one morning around her due date and did not think much of the contractions until, at about 8am, she was taken aback by suddenly much stronger contractions. She found what looked like water mixed with blood trickling down her thighs and phoned me immediately, thinking she was bleeding.

I was at her side within 10 minutes and, on examination, found she was fully dilated and ready to push. She was so surprised I gave her some Rescue Remedy to ease the shock of finding out things had progressed so rapidly. As there was no time to fill the birthing pool, I ran a bath for her and she sat in the warm water and gave birth just as the community midwives arrived. The recorded time of her entire labour, that she was aware of, was two hours.

Haemorrhoids (Piles)

What are they?: Piles are engorged veins that are located in the lowest part of the rectum, just within the anal canal. However, they can sometimes protrude. These veins are areas where the portal veins (intestinal veins) join the general veins from the rest of the body.

What causes them?: Increased pressure from the pregnant uterus on the pelvic veins can result in back pressure on the matrix of veins around the rectum and cause a simple dilatation of the piles (venous engorgement). Constipation can also increase this pressure at the region of the piles and cause an engorgement. Other causes of piles include portal hypertension i.e. when there is an inability of the gut veins to drain through the liver through narrowing of the bilary veins. This more serious condition is not usually associated with pregnancy, and is observed in cirrhosis of the liver.

How can they be alleviated?:

- Creative Healing: A specific treatment on the coccyx and sacral area is very efficient in reducing them. (See page 214 in the Post-natal section for a description of how to do this movement.)
- Ayurveda: The Ayurvedic method of treating piles is to wear a sanitary towel that has been soaked in warm olive oil and then lie down on a plastic mat, ensuring the pad is in contact with your piles, for an hour a day – a wonderful remedy!
- A sitz bath may be helpful. Sit in a bath with 15cm (6in) of body-temperature water and 20 drops of cypress essential oil.
- Cold compresses for 20 minutes, 3 times a day, can assist with the discomfort.
- Make sure that you can empty your bowels easily, so eat more vegetables and drink plenty of water.
- If you are constantly constipated you may need to use a mild glycerine suppository to help ease the movement of your bowels.
- Homoeopathic remedies: (all remedies below, unless otherwise indicated, should be taken twice a day for 3–4 days)
  - Hamamelis 30c, good for piles that occur towards the end of pregnancy and childbirth – especially useful if piles are associated with bleeding, soreness and bruising

- Nux vom. 6c, three times a day for four days, for sensitive inflamed piles that are associated with constipation and that feel worse at night
- Ignatia 30c, good for internal piles that cause shooting pains and that seem to manifest after childbirth – usually associated with anxiousness in pregnancy
- Sepia 30c can help with constipation associated with piles

Overdue Baby

What is it?: When pregnancy progresses beyond 38–42 weeks.

What causes it?: A common cause is maternal anxiety about birth. It has been noted that in stressful situations, for instance in war zones, mothers have a longer gestation. Physical causes include a uterus that is unresponsive to oxytocin, and diabetes mellitus. Molecular biologists have identified that a sufficient number of cell-membrane receptors need to develop in order for oestrogen and oxytocin to work in a coordinated manner during labour. If there are fewer cell-membrane receptors, even if sufficient doses of oxytocin are given to the uterus, the uterine muscles are unable to respond. Nutritional deficiencies may contribute to the lack of sufficient numbers of cell-membrane receptors forming.

How can you encourage labour?:

- Dietary supplements. To ensure that nutritional deficiencies do not cause the baby to be overdue, the following dietary supplements are advised: essential fatty acids (omega 3, 6 and 9); essential sugars; and anti-oxidants (e.g. vitamins C and E), found in general prenatal vitamin and mineral tablets or capsules. For further information on these supplements see the box on Omega 3 and 'Nutritional and Herbal Supplements', Section A, pages 10–11. (For stockist details see Appendix C, pages 311–12.) Note: if you had an overdue baby previously, or babies going over their due dates are common in your family, then it is highly recommended that you take these dietary supplements.
- Reflexology can be used as a trigger to initiate labour by applying very strong pressure to the pituitary, adrenal and uterine area. A complete reflexology treatment to relax the mother is also helpful.

- Exercise can stimulate labour at term, especially if there have been a few mild contractions that indicate pre-labour. Try a long (40 minute), brisk walk. The walking motion enables the baby's head to bear down on the cervix, encouraging dilatation.
- Nipple stimulation is known to release oxytocin from your posterior pituitary gland and can bring on contractions.
- Sex: It is known that semen contains prostaglandins, the medical agents used to induce labour. Therefore sex can be a more natural method of introducing prostaglandins into your vagina – and as well as helping to initiate labour, they will soften the cervix.
- Listening to the Birth Rehearsal tape and/or the Jeyarani Labour tape can overcome subconscious fears about birth.
- Homoeopathic remedies: (choose the most appropriate remedies below, take one a day for 2 days then have a 2-day break and before trying again)
  - Caulophyllum 200c, this is known to thin out the cervix
  - Aconite 200c, if there are subconscious fears of birth and maybe palpitations
  - Gelsemium 200c, if there is an anticipatory anxiety of labour and maybe looseness of the bowels

Piles (see Haemorrhoids, page 261)

Placental Abruption

What is it?: Abnormal, premature separation of a normally located placenta. If separation is over a small area, this clots and heals and there may be minimal symptoms. A pregnant mother who has a bleed needs to be instantly investigated because of the dangers of the baby not getting enough oxygen, which can lead to foetal distress and maybe stillbirth. Even minor degrees of suspected placental abruption necessitate that the growth of the baby is monitored at regular intervals using ultra-sound scans because small areas of the placenta could become non-functional due to clots, thereby impeding the baby's development.

If the placenta separates over a larger area there can be abdominal pain with vaginal bleeding. Sometimes, however, the blood does not actually leak out and is contained in the placental bed. The mother then develops lower abdominal pain, rapidly followed by a rapid drop in the blood pressure, so she may feel cold and clammy. If the abdominal pain is severe enough then the mother should go immediately to hospital. In severe placental abruption the mother can become unconsciousness.

What causes it?: Usually there is no obvious cause, but vitamin and mineral deficiencies and deficiencies of essential fatty acids, sugars and proteins (amino acids) can contribute to poor capillary integrity in the placental bed. Rarely, trauma and direct impact can cause bleeding from the placenta. If there is a deficiency of clotting factors in the blood there can be a predisposition to bleeding.

Important note:
- If you can see vaginal bleeding *lie still* (movement can increase bleeding) and call for help and an ambulance straightaway. If you feel faint, lie down and elevate your legs as high as you can on several sets of pillows to keep up your blood pressure.

How can it be prevented?:
- Prevention is always better than cure and I am a great advocate of a pre-conception programme of a good diet and supplements to provide all the necessary vitamins, minerals, trace elements, high-quality antioxidants and essential fatty acids, sugars and amino acids. This is in line with several organizations, like Foresight, who promote pre-conceptual care to assist fertility. Tissue integrity at implantation ensures a strong placental bed, thereby preventing these sorts of complications. The Gentle Birth Method promotes nutritional support all the way through pregnancy to strengthen blood vessels and capillaries in your whole body, including the uterus and placenta.

Important note: clinical care only. Contact your GP or midwife. Once you have had a clinical assessment, try the homoeopathic remedies to reduce shock.

- Take 4 drops of Bach Flower Rescue Remedy on your tongue instantly to calm you down.
- Homoeopathic remedies:
  - Aconite 30c as a single dose can ease your fear as a first-aid remedy
  - Arnica 30c as a single dose can help ease the pain, until you get to hospital

Placenta Praevia
What is it?: The implantation of the placenta low in the uterus, so that it encroaches on the cervix and the lower segment of the uterus. The lower segment only usually develops after 32 weeks of pregnancy. Therefore if an early scan shows that your placenta is encroaching on the lower segment, if you are lucky, after 32 weeks, it will grow up and away from the internal cervical opening.

There are four grades of Placenta Praevia:
Grade I – the edge of the placenta encroaches on the lower segment, but does not reach the internal opening of the cervix into the uterus
Grade II – the placenta's edge reaches into the internal opening of the cervix, but does not cover it
Grade III – the placenta partly covers the internal opening of the cervix
Grade IV – the placenta completely covers the internal opening of the cervix

In all grades of Placenta Praevia there may be bouts of bleeding throughout pregnancy and labour, and post-partum haemorrhage. Vaginal delivery may be possible in Grades I and II if there has not been any bleeding. However, a caesarean is necessary to deliver the baby of grades III and IV, as the baby cannot descend into the vagina. If labour commences, there is a chance of torrential haemorrhage occurring, which is life-threatening.
What causes it?: Implantation of the placenta can occur on the anterior, posterior and lateral walls of the cervix, and is entirely random. Commonly, poor tone and laxity of the uterine muscle wall has been implicated as one of the causes of Placenta Praevia. It is therefore more common in mothers who

have had many pregnancies, causing the uterine muscle wall to be over-stretched. Pre-conceptual nutrition is very important to strengthen the uterine muscles for optimum implantation so if you are planning a pregnancy ensure you take general vitamin and mineral supplements. I also recommend that you take Ambrotose to ensure that you get the 8 essential sugars (this can be obtained from Jeyarani, see Appendix C, page 312). The essential fats (omega 3, 6 and 9) are also important (see omega 3 box on page 10).

Important note: Routine ultra-sound scans are invaluable in picking up abnormal implantations of the placenta. In all grades of Placenta Praevia a watchful eye needs to be maintained by the mother and clinician in charge, which will necessitate admission to hospital. In most cases mothers seem to be happily symptom-free until the later stages of pregnancy. Hopefully, if the mother can get to 32 weeks, the baby will be viable and ready for delivery by caesarean at the earliest sign of bleeding. Reams can be written about the obstetric management of Placenta Praevia, please consult an appropriate textbook for more detailed information.

How can it be alleviated?:
• Creative Healing: With grades I and II, abdominal toning and pelvic drainage can help the placenta to grow up and away from the cervix. If you've got Placenta Praevia please see a Creative healer, do not do this at home because the touch needs to be extremely light.
• Reiki can provide emotional support.
• Do not have reflexology if you have grades III and IV. Those with grades I and II can have light reflexology only, avoiding the reflex areas of the uterus and pituitary gland.
• Homoeopathic remedies: Consult a homoeopath. Once you have been diagnosed with any degree of Placenta Praevia your homoeopath will help to minimize sudden bleeding or any damage to your uterus and cervix.

Pregnancy-induced Hypertension (Pre-eclampsia)

What is it?: Raised blood pressure, associated with fluid retention and proteins present in the urine – a symptom complex known as Pre-eclampsia. Mild eclampsia occurs in 5 per cent of first pregnancies. It seems to occur more after 32 weeks of pregnancy. Normal blood pressure is in the range of 120/80 to 140/90 mm of mercury. In mild pre-eclampsia blood pressure can go up to 140/100 with associated swelling of the feet or hands. The urine is usually clear. However, in severe cases, blood pressure may go above 160/110 and there may be protein loss in the urine. Symptoms of pre-eclampsia may include headaches, dizziness and in severe cases blurred vision, irritability, nausea and even fits. There is a marked reduction in blood flow to the placenta and this can lead to foetal hypoxia (reduction of oxygen supply to the baby) in late pregnancy and especially during labour, bringing an increased risk of stillbirth. The baby may also suffer intrauterine growth retardation and have a low birth weight. Risks to the mother include the condition developing into Eclampsia (see page 257).

What causes it?: The reasons are obscure but could be linked to stress or poor nutrition.

How can it be alleviated?:

- Creative Healing: The General treatment (see pages 55–64), which is also a lymphatic drainage applied to the neck and upper back, is *the* treatment for high blood pressure. If the blood pressure is more than 160/110, apply the General treatment every day for 20 minutes for 4 days in a row. Supportive treatments are heart treatment and kidney treatment done on the first day of the course of treatments. See a Creative healer for advice.
- Reflexology is particularly good at relieving stress and anxiety and normalizing blood pressure. Ask for an all-round treatment with emphasis on the head and neck, kidney and adrenal areas.
- Cranio-sacral therapy can help by treating the focal point of cerebral stress.
- Bowen treatment can help by having a profoundly sedating effect.
- Homoeopathic remedies: Consult a homoeopath.

Pubic Pain

What is it?: A pain in the region of the pubic bone at the lowest part of the abdomen where the hip bones meet at a central point. Stresses and strains of the growing uterus pressing upon that area, coupled with sprained lower abdominal muscles, can contribute to this pain.

What causes it?: This usually occurs in the later half of pregnancy due to the increasing size of the baby. The pregnancy hormones also soften the muscles and can cause the muscles to be easily pulled by sudden movements. On occasion this pain can be caused by separation of the joint of the symphysis pubis (see Symphysis Pubis Diastasis, page 271).

How can it be alleviated?:

- In severe cases, rest and anti-inflammatories may be prescribed.
- Cranial-osteopaths and general osteopaths are good at treating this condition.
- Acupuncture.
- Reflexology can help by increasing the lymphatic drainage and by decongesting the area. Reflexology also releases endorphins, which are natural painkillers.
- Creative Healing: Pelvic drainage treatment (see pages 68–9). A full sciatic treatment can help. See a Creative healer for advice.
- Bowen is particularly good at treating acute pelvic pain as it can be applied even when muscles are very sore.
- Homoeopathic remedies:
  - Rhus tox. 30c twice a day for 3 days

Clinical Notes: Pubic pain in pregnancy
Helen, 32 years old, first pregnancy

At 36-weeks gestation, Helen presented with pubic pain. I examined her pelvis and found it to be tilted and with muscle spasm in her lower lumbar area.

In one session, I gave her a 20-minute Creative Healing treatment to decongest and relax the back muscles and reposition displaced substance along the inter-vertebral spaces. I also worked on the sacrum to decongest the ligaments overlying the sacro-iliac joints, and put back the nerve centre between the second and third piece of the sacrum on the midline.

I followed this up with a 15-minute Bowen technique to release the buttock muscles, the quadriceps, hamstrings, the inguinal ligament, the pelvic muscles and the sacrum and coccyx.

No follow up treatment was necessary and Helen was pleased and surprised that one treatment was sufficient to relieve her pubic pain.

Restless legs (also see Restless Legs Syndrome in The Second Trimester, page 250)

What is it?: An involuntary twitching of the legs caused by spontaneous and unpleasant neuro-muscular responses. It can come on suddenly in pregnancy and is not a serious condition.

What causes it?: It can be associated with anxiety and dietary deficiencies, though more commonly the cause cannot be identified.

How can it be alleviated?:
• Nutrition: Take a general pregnancy vitamin and mineral supplement (see Appendix C, pages 311–312) as these contain vitamins and minerals that support the central nervous system.

- You can have your B12 levels tested by your GP by a blood test and if found to be deficient your GP will prescribe accordingly.
- Homoeopathic remedies:
  - Zinc 30c once a day for 3 days – if there is no improvement refer to a homoeopath
  - Follow the Homoeopathic Tissue Salt Programme (sees pages 12–13)

Swollen Ankles (oedema)

What is it?: Fluid retention in the lower legs, illustrated by a loss of muscular definition around the ankle area.

What causes it?: There can be a number of causes – incompetent venous return to the heart; pelvic vein congestion caused by the pregnant uterus sitting heavily on the pelvic vein; and protein loss in urine causing hypoproteinaemia in the general circulation (pre-eclamptic toxaemia).

How can it be alleviated?:

- Reflexology: A treatment focusing on lymphatic drainage, i.e. working on the tops of the feet in the thoracic drainage areas along with the pelvic drainage areas will be helpful. Stimulating the kidneys and the intestines will also be of great benefit.
- Creative healing: Abdominal toning (see pages 67–8) and Pelvic drainage (see pages 68–9).
- Homoeopathic remedies: (for each of the remedies below take once a day for 3 days)
  - Zinc 30c
  - Apis Mellifica 6c – can be used to reduce swellings in ankles/feet or hands/fingers that are shiny and rosy-red in colour. This may be accompanied by restlessness
  - Nat. Mur. 30c when swelling is accompanied by a desire for salt, and thirst
  - Follow the Homoeopathic Tissue Salt Programme (sees pages 12–13)

Symphysis Pubis Diastasis

What is it?: The joints between the two pubic bones (symphysis pubis) begin to separate, resulting in severe pain at the front of the pelvis, radiating into the groin and vaginal wall. In severe cases, postural stability is lost hence the mother is unable to walk and has to use a wheelchair.

What causes it?: The effect of the increased amounts of progesterone circulating around the body in this instance drastically relaxes the muscles in the pubic joints, leaving them unable to support the weight of the pregnant uterus, hence they begin to separate.

How can it be alleviated?:

- Analgesics.
- Anti-inflammatories.
- Reflexology: A deep general treatment concentrating on lymphatic drainage in the pelvic and hip joint areas will help.
- Creative Healing: Have a General treatment and then pelvic drainage in the lower part of the front abdomen. Your partner can perform General treatment (see pages 55–64) and pelvic drainage (see pages 68–9); see practitioner for specific sciatic treatment if necessary.
- Bowen: A treatment that includes all the core level Bowen moves with specific pelvic release techniques has proved extremely effective.
- Homoeopathic remedies:
  - Arnica 30c helps the pain and is useful when you feel bruised – take twice a day for 3 days
  - Symphytum 30c, the common term for it is 'bone knit', has been to known to help – take twice a day for 3 days

Thrombosis (deep leg vein)

What is it?: A clot that develops in the major veins. It can be life-threatening if a thrombosis fragments and travels to the lungs.

What causes it?: Increased coagulability of the blood during pregnancy, due to raised fibrinogen levels in circulation. Periods of inactivity can also encourage blood circulation to become sluggish, resulting in compression of the vein.

Dehydration can also cause this condition.

Important note:
- Any painful calf complaint should be investigated – if serious, you will require hospitalization and anti-coagulant therapy.
- See your GP immediately.

How can it be alleviated?:
- Creative Healing as first aid: Use your cupped hands, coated in olive oil, to create a cooling breeze, drawing downwards in a kind of stroking movement – note that your hands should not touch the skin and your palms should face the leg that you are treating (see page 54).
- Homoeopathic remedies:
  - Consult a homoeopath
  - Arnica 200c, four hourly during the daytime for 2–3 days until the pain subsides. It is an anti-inflammatory and good for pain-relief
  - Kali. Mur. 6c, four times a day for 7 days. This is an alternative option.

Varicose Veins
What is it?: Enlargement of the vein, most commonly found in the legs (behind the knee) and the vulva.
What causes it?: The weight of the pregnant uterus contributes to the back pressure on the veins, causing swelling and enlargement.

How can it be alleviated?:
- Wear support stockings at the first sign of varicose veins.
- Do not sit with your legs crossed.
- Creative Healing: Using both hands, *lightly* massage the legs in a *downward* direction using virgin olive oil. Your hands should be open and cupped. The intention is to gently drain the legs. Start from mid-thigh and go to the ankles. This should be done repeatedly for 5 minutes on each leg. Do NOT go in an upward direction.
- Encourage good circulation in the area by applying topical stimulants such

as peppermint cream.
- Aid circulation and drainage of the area by drinking lots of water.
- Do not stand for long periods of time.
- Try to rest with your feet above your heart at least once a day for 15 minutes. Try lying on the floor with your legs straight above you and fully supported against a wall. Place a cushion under your head and shoulders.
- Homoeopathic remedies:
  - Ferr. Met. 6c for swollen and painful varicosities in leg, thigh and foot, particularly if it is worse at night when at rest – one dose four times a day for 4 days
  - Hamamelis 6c for veins that are painful, bruised and sore; also if swollen and inflamed with hard and knotty varicosities – four times a day for 4 days
  - Pulsatilla 6c for painful veins; also if worse with warmth and when sitting down with hanging down limbs – four times a day for 5 days
  - Bryonia or Calc. Carb. 6c for vulval varicosities – one dose twice a day for 3 days (Bryonia is indicated if it is worse with movement)

APPENDICES

Appendix A

Gentle Birth Method Recipes

These recipes are all tridoshic, which means that all mothers, regardless of their dosha predominance, can enjoy them. Even better, you don't have to be pregnant to eat them – so the whole family can tuck in too!

Ghee

Ghee is a basic component of many Ayurvedic dishes. While sunflower oil or butter can be used as an alternative, ghee is far superior in its properties and digestibility. It acts as a body purifier that absorbs and expels toxins from the body. As it doesn't have even a trace of milk solids, it can be stored for quite a long time.

225g (8oz) unsalted butter
4 whole cloves

Place the butter in a saucepan and let it melt over a medium heat until the foam rises to the surface. Take care not to burn it. Add the cloves – these not only provide a delicate flavour but also help to clarify the butter.

Turn down the heat to low and cook, uncovered, until the milk solids collect on the bottom of the pan and turn a golden colour. Using a large spoon, skim off any crust that rises to the surface and discard it.

The ghee is the golden liquid above the milk solids at the bottom of the pan. Ladle off the ghee and put it in a clean container to cool. Be careful not to disturb the milk solids at the bottom of the pan.

The ghee in the container is now ready to use.

Lunches

Chicken and Vegetable Soup *(Serves 4)*

1 tbsp ghee or olive oil
1 medium onion, chopped
4 medium parsnips, peeled and chopped
2 carrots, chopped
1 leek, sliced
1 litre (1¾ pints) vegetable stock (can be made with bouillon powder or
 vegetable stock cubes)
2 large, boned and skinned chicken breasts, cut into bite-sized pieces
1 tbsp mild mustard
Salt and freshly ground black pepper
Freshly grated nutmeg
2 tbsp fromage frais
Fresh coriander leaves to garnish

Heat the ghee or oil in a large saucepan, add the chopped onion and sauté until it is lightly brown.

Add the remaining vegetables to the pan and cook over a medium heat until the vegetables glisten – about 20 minutes.

Add the stock to the saucepan and bring to the boil. Reduce the heat and simmer the soup until the vegetables are soft.

Remove from the heat, stir in the chopped chicken and mustard and cook gently for 15 minutes until the chicken is fully cooked.

Season with salt, pepper and nutmeg. Stir in the fromage frais and garnish with coriander before serving.

Avocado Spread *(Serves 2)*

This healthy spread is delicious as part of a wheat-free sandwich, and because it is moist there is no need for butter or margarine. (This is nice on soda bread, see page 297.)

    1 ripe avocado
    1 tbsp lime or lemon juice
    1 tbsp chopped fresh coriander leaves
    ⅛ tsp garlic powder or a little fresh crushed garlic, or from a tube
    ⅛ tsp fresh ground black pepper

Mash all the ingredients together in a small bowl using a fork. Serve on corn bread, rice cakes or corn crispbreads and enjoy!

Scrambled Tofu *(Serves 2)*

This is excellent on wheat-free toast such as soda bread (see page 297).

    1 tbsp ghee or butter
    ¼ tsp mustard seeds
    225g (½ lb) tofu
    ¼ tsp turmeric
    ¼ tsp black pepper
    ¼ tsp rock or sea salt
    A pinch of ground cumin

Warm the ghee or butter in a saucepan. When the butter is melted, add the mustard seeds and heat until they begin to pop.

Add the tofu and mash it into small pieces with a fork or potato masher.

Add the rest of the ingredients and stir well. Cook for 3–5 minutes on a medium heat then serve.

Main Dishes

Kitchidi *(Serves 2)*

Kitchidi is a nourishing, balancing meal containing rice, mung dhal and spices. It is easy to digest and is a healthy alternative to wheat-based meals. You can eat it 3–4 times a week – and you'll want to, it really is delicious!

> 200g (7oz) basmati rice
> 100g (3½ oz) mung dhal
> *Note: the above 2 ingredients need to be washed and then soaked together in water for at least 4–6 hours or overnight*
> 2 tbsp ghee (or olive oil)
> ¼ tsp mustard seeds
> 1 tsp chopped fresh ginger root
> 1 garlic clove, crushed
> 4 peppercorns
> 4 cloves
> 2 cardamom pods
> ¼ tsp turmeric
> 500ml (18fl oz) water
> Salt to taste
> Fresh coriander to garnish – optional

Place the ghee or olive oil in a large pan and warm gently until it has melted.

Add the mustard seeds and when they begin to crackle slightly, add the ginger and garlic and sauté for 1–2 minutes.

Now add the peppercorns, cloves and cardamom pods (make sure these are split open a little to allow the flavour to escape) and sauté for a further 2–3 minutes.

Drain the soaked rice and dhal, add them to the pan and heat, stirring occasionally, for 1–2 minutes.

Add the turmeric and then the water, stirring thoroughly. Add salt to taste.

Partially cover the pan and heat the Kitchidi over a very gentle heat for 15–20 minutes.

Once cooked it can be served with chopped coriander leaves as a garnish.

Quinoa with Vegetables *(Serves 6)*

Quinoa can be bought from larger supermarkets or healthfood stores.

140g (5oz) uncooked quinoa
500ml (18fl oz) water
2 tsp olive oil
2 medium onions, chopped
1 large red or green pepper, chopped
1 large garlic clove, crushed
300g (10 oz) pack frozen vegetables (this is a timesaving option – you can substitute with your choice of sautéed vegetables)
¼ tsp salt
⅛ tsp ground black pepper
1 tbsp chopped coriander

Rinse the quinoa in a strainer under running water and drain.

Place the quinoa and the water in a saucepan and bring to the boil. Reduce the heat and simmer, stirring occasionally, until the quinoa is translucent

(10–15 minutes). Let it stand for 10 minutes. Drain, if necessary.

Meanwhile, heat the oil over medium heat in a large frying pan. Add the chopped onion and pepper and cook, stirring often, for about 5 minutes until crisp-tender.

Add the garlic and cook, stirring constantly, for 30 seconds.

Add the mixed vegetables, salt and pepper, and cook, stirring often, for about 5 minutes until vegetables are tender-crisp.

Add the coriander and cooked quinoa and heat thoroughly.

Asparagus and Goat's Cheese Salad *(Serves 2)*

N.B. Goat's cheese is tridoshic and does not aggravate any dosha.

> 225g (½lb) asparagus
> A little olive oil
> 85g (3oz) toasted walnuts
> 100g (3½oz) ripe goat's cheese, sliced
> A pinch of dried mixed herbs
> 1 crisp cos lettuce, washed and sliced
> A handful of fresh watercress
> A handful of fresh basil leaves
> ½ tsp lime juice
> Salt and freshly ground black pepper

Preheat oven to 200°C/400°F/Gas mark 6.

Trim the woody ends off the asparagus. Brush the asparagus with a little olive oil and place them on a non-stick baking tray. Roast in the oven for about 15 minutes until tender.

Spread the walnuts in an oil-free frying pan and dry-fry them until golden. Place the roasted nuts in a bowl.

Season the goat's cheese with the mixed herbs.

Arrange the lettuce and watercress on two plates. Place the hot asparagus on the salad leaves and sprinkle over the nuts.

Quickly grill the goat's cheese until each piece is warm and slightly melting in the centre. Place the cheese on the salad, sprinkle over the basil leaves and lime juice and season with salt and pepper to taste.

Garlicky Haddock *(Serves 4)*

4 medium-sized boneless and skinless thick fillets of fresh haddock
4 tbsp olive oil
2 heaped tbsp whole almonds
1 handful blanched parsley
1 garlic clove, crushed
A pinch of sea salt
Freshly ground black pepper

Preheat the oven to 200°C/400°F/Gas mark 6.

Lay the haddock fillets in a shallow baking dish (one that can also be used for serving).

Put all the other ingredients into a blender and blend to a finely chopped sauce. Spread this sauce over the top of the fish and bake in the oven for about 20 minutes (the fish should be cooked through and the sauce will have browned slightly).

Serve the fish in the dish accompanied by a salad or steamed vegetables.

Note: Cod or salmon can be used as an alternative to haddock.

Mackerel with Vegetables *(Serves 2)*

Mackerel is packed with omega-3 fatty acids.

1 tbsp olive oil
1 small onion

1 bowl of thinly sliced carrots, leeks, parsnips and 1 tomato
Freshly ground pepper
2 mackerel, cleaned
Salt
Pinch of dried mixed herbs
15g (½ oz) fresh chives, chopped

Heat the oil in a frying pan and cook the onions for about 8 minutes until they are soft.

Stir in the vegetables, season with pepper, add enough water to facilitate cooking and simmer gently for about 10–15 minutes. Stir occasionally, adding a little water as necessary.

Meanwhile, preheat the grill then sprinkle the fish with a little salt and the herbs and grill them for about 10 minutes until they are cooked through and the skin is crisp. (Do not turn them over.)

Place the mackerel on top of the vegetables and sprinkle with the chopped chives.

Cod and Courgette Bake *(Serves 2)*

As an alternative to cod, salmon, haddock, swordfish, skate wings or monkfish are delicious. You can also use vegetables according to your preference – for instance, green beans (put the beans in boiling water for 1 minute before roasting them) or sweet peppers.

2 cod fillets
1 tbsp light soy sauce
Juice of ½ a lemon
Salt
Freshly ground black pepper
1 large onion
2 large fennel bulbs

Olive oil
4 medium tomatoes
225g (½ lb) courgettes
1 tsp mixed herbs
Handful of chopped fresh parsley to garnish

For the dressing:
1 tsp clear honey
2 tbsp balsamic vinegar (avoid if pitta is high)
2 tbsp olive oil
1 heaped tsp mild mustard
1 garlic clove, crushed
Salt
Freshly ground black pepper

Mix all ingredients for the dressing in a bowl and set aside.

Preheat the oven to 200°C/400°F/Gas mark 6.

Place the cod fillets in an ovenproof dish, sprinkle with soy sauce and lemon juice and season with a little salt and pepper. Set aside for 30 minutes.

Trim, peel and cut the onion and fennel into chunks. Put the onion and fennel into a big non-stick roasting tin, brush with a little olive oil and sprinkle with the mixed herbs and some pepper. Roast in the oven for about 10–15 minutes, until they are beginning to soften. Remove from the oven.

Now place the cod in the oven and bake for 15 minutes.

Cut the courgettes into diagonal slices of about 2cm thick. Add the courgettes and whole tomatoes to the fennel and onions in the roasting tin, drizzle with a little extra olive oil and place the tin back in the oven for 10 minutes.

Serve the fish straightaway with the roasted vegetables and dressing. Sprinkle with chopped parsley if desired.

Note: Any leftover dressing should be kept in a sealed container at room temperature.

Sardines on Wheat-free Toast *(Serves 2)*

8 fresh sardines, cleaned
Salt and freshly ground black pepper
1 tbsp olive oil
1 small garlic clove, crushed
Pinch of dried mixed herbs
2 large slices Soda Bread (see page 297) or any other type of
     wheat-free bread
½ tsp lemon juice
1 tbsp chopped fresh parsley to garnish

Preheat the grill for 5 minutes on maximum.

Sprinkle the sardines with salt, pepper, oil, garlic and herbs and heat under the grill until they are cooked through.

Meanwhile, make the toast.

Place the sardines across the toast, squeeze some lemon juice on top and garnish with the parsley.

Roast Chicken with Tarragon

A medium-sized chicken will usually serve 4

1 corn-fed, free-range, organic chicken
3 onions, quartered
Fresh tarragon
2 tbsp olive oil
1 tsp salt
1 tsp crushed peppercorns
2 tsp dried herbs
2 garlic cloves, sliced

Preheat the oven to 180°C/350°F/Gas mark 4.

Place the chicken in a roasting dish and arrange the quartered onions and some tarragon around it.

Drizzle over the olive oil and sprinkle on the salt, crushed peppercorns, dried herbs and the slices of garlic.

Cook in the oven for 20 minutes per 400g – a 1.35kg/3lb chicken will therefore take about 70 minutes. Check the chicken is cooked by piercing the thigh with a skewer – if the juices run clear it is ready.

Vegetable Side Dishes

In general, vegetables rule. They're rich in vitamins and low in calories and, when they're properly prepared, they are amongst the easiest foods to digest. You can have vegetables with most foods, including fats, proteins and grains.

Asparagus, parsnips, artichokes, okra, green beans and string beans are well tolerated by all doshas. According to Ayurvedic medicine, asparagus is particularly useful as it has a mild laxative effect, it calms the nerves, is a general tonic, an aphrodisiac and it helps reduce mucus. As well as being a tasty addition to some of the following recipes, it's great simply steamed and served with a little ghee.

Asparagus and Parsnips *(Serves 4–5)*

This dish goes well with rice.

> 455g (1lb) fresh asparagus
> 3 medium parsnips
> 1–2 tbsp sunflower oil or ghee
> ¼ tsp black mustard seeds
> ½ tsp turmeric
> 125ml (4fl oz) water

1 tbsp ground coriander
½ tsp sea salt
⅓ tsp ground cumin
A few crushed peppercorns

Cut the asparagus into 2.5cm (1in) pieces. Peel the parsnips and cut into 1.5cm (½in) cubes.

Put half of the oil into a large saucepan, place on a medium heat and add the mustard seeds. When the mustard seeds pop, stir in the turmeric, chopped asparagus and parsnips. Mix well.

Add the water and the rest of the ingredients and cover the pan. Cook over a medium heat for about 4 minutes.

Now turn the heat down and cook for another 8–10 minutes.

If you don't fancy asparagus today, then substitute 455g (1lb) of green beans. Alternatively, try a mixture of okra and potatoes. Use 455g (1lb) fresh okra instead of the asparagus and 2 small potatoes instead of the parsnips.

Green Bhaji *(Serves 4)*

This vegetable dish goes well with dhal and rice.

455g (1lb) fresh green beans (the fresher the better)
1 tbsp sunflower oil or ghee
½ tsp black mustard seeds
1 tsp turmeric
5–7 tbsp water
½ tsp sea salt
3 tbsp chopped fresh coriander leaves
2.5cm (1in) piece fresh ginger root, chopped
1 small fresh green chilli (pitta mothers should omit this)
Chopped fresh coriander leaves to garnish

Wash the green beans and cut into 5cm (2in) strips.

Warm the oil or ghee in a large saucepan. Add the mustard seeds and cook until they start to pop.

Add the turmeric, stirring well.

Add the chopped green beans and 2–3 tablespoons of water. Cover with a lid and cook on a low heat for 15–30 minutes until the beans are tender.

Put 3–4 tablespoons of water and the remaining ingredients (salt, coriander, ginger and chilli) in a blender and purée.

Pour the purée into the saucepan, over the cooked beans, and mix well. Simmer for 1–2 minutes.

Garnish with coriander if desired.

Lovely Dark Leafy Greens *(Serves 2–3)*

Use dark leafy greens such as chicory, kale and turnip greens for this dish – they are excellent and can be eaten freely.

    1 bunch of dark leafy greens e.g. kale
    125–200ml (4–7fl oz) water
    1 tsp sunflower oil or ghee
    ½ tsp whole cumin seeds
    1 tsp ground coriander

Wash and chop the greens. Use the tender parts only.

Bring the water to the boil in a large saucepan and add the chopped greens. Cover the pan and simmer for 7–15 minutes until the greens are tender.

Meanwhile, heat the oil in a frying pan. Add the cumin seeds and when they begin to brown, stir in the coriander. Keep the heat low so that you don't burn this mixture.

Drain the greens. (You can save this water to make a soup if desired; other people like to drink it like tea in a cup!)

Now pour the oil, cumin and coriander mixture over the drained greens and mix well. Serve and eat straightaway – they really are, as they're called, 'lovely'!

Popular Potatoes *(Serves 2–3)*

Potatoes can be eaten on this programme in moderation (ensure that any green areas are completely cut out), however, the way they are cooked is very important to determine whether they are acceptable to a particular dosha. All dosha types can enjoy this recipe.

> 8 new potatoes with skins
> 125ml (4fl oz) goat's milk, hot (or rice milk)
> 4 tbsp sunflower oil or ghee (vata mothers can use more ghee)
> 1 tsp sea salt
> 1 tsp chopped fresh tarragon
> 1 tbsp chopped fresh parsley or coriander leaves (optional)

Put enough water to cover the potatoes in a pan and bring to the boil.

Wash the potatoes and when the water is boiling, add them to the pan. Boil the potatoes for about 20 minutes until tender.

Drain and put the potatoes in a large bowl.

Mash the potatoes with a fork or masher, stirring in the hot goat's milk and ghee as you mash.

Season with salt, and add the tarragon and the parsley or coriander as desired.

Smashing Squash *(Serves 3–4)*

> 1 large yellow butternut (or similar) squash
> 3 tbsp ghee or butter (only 1 tbsp if kapha predominant)
> ½ small onion, chopped

      1 garlic clove, unpeeled
      1 tbsp chopped fresh parsley
      1 tsp chopped fresh dill (or ½ tsp dried dill)
      ½ tsp sea salt
      A few crushed peppercorns

Chop the squash into cubes.

Warm the ghee or butter in a large pan. Add the onion and unpeeled garlic to the pan and sauté for 2–3 minutes.

Add the squash and cook, uncovered, over a medium heat for about 5–10 minutes until tender.

Add all the other ingredients, cover and cook for another 10 minutes, stirring occasionally.

Remove the garlic before serving.

Courgettes and Herbs *(Serves 3–4)*

      2 medium courgettes
      2 tbsp sunflower oil
      125ml (4fl oz) water
      ½ tsp turmeric
      1 bunch fresh dill or coriander leaves, chopped
      2 tbsp lemon juice
      1 tbsp maple syrup
      1½ tsp ground coriander

Slice the courgettes into slices about 2cm (¾ in) thick.

Heat the oil in a pan. Add the water, courgettes and turmeric.

Cover the pan and cook for 5 minutes.

Add the rest of the ingredients and cook for a further 5 minutes.

Gowri's Courgettes *(Serves 2)*

1 tbsp olive oil
¼ tsp mustard seeds
1 garlic clove, crushed
2 small courgettes, sliced
¼ tsp turmeric
Chopped fresh dill to garnish

Heat the olive oil in a non-stick frying pan. When hot, add the mustard seeds. When they begin to pop, add the garlic and stir for 1 minute.

Now add the courgettes and turmeric and sauté for 3 minutes, stirring often. Serve the cooked courgettes garnished with the dill.

Desserts

Here are a few simple recipes that should help satisfy the occasional desire for something sweet – but without breaking the dietary guidelines on what is healthy for you and your baby.

All mothers, regardless of their predominant dosha, can eat three fruits a day. Berries, cherries and apricots can be enjoyed – but only one small bowl per day. You can have two slices of fresh pineapple per day (it's good for digestion) but only as one of your three portions of fruit. Apples and pears can be stewed or baked to suit all doshas. Dried figs can be stewed and served plain for pitta and vata.

Fresh Fruit Salad *(Serves 3–4)*

115g (4oz) strawberries, hulled
115g (4oz) fresh apricots, halved and stoned
115g (4oz) blueberries or raspberries

1 tbsp lemon juice
1 tbsp maple syrup
Fresh mint leaves (optional)

If the strawberries are large, chop them into small pieces.

Put all the fruit into a serving bowl. Drizzle the juice and maple syrup over the fruit and mix well.

Serve with a garnish of mint leaves if desired.

Stewed Apricots *(Serves 2–3)*

340g (12oz) dried apricots
500ml (18fl oz) water
250ml (9fl oz) unsweetened apple juice
1 tsp lemon juice (optional)
2.5cm (1in) piece of cinnamon stick

Put all the ingredients in a saucepan, place over a medium heat and simmer until the apricots are tender. Serve hot or cold.

Fabulous Figs (or Perfect Prunes) *(Serves 2)*

This is a simple but delicious snack for when your energy levels run low.

225g (8oz) dried figs or prunes
500ml (18fl oz) boiling water

Place the figs or prunes in a glass bowl. Pour boiling water over the fruit and let it soak for about 15 minutes. Enjoy!

Super Spicy Pears *(Serves 4)*

5 dried apricots
5 ripe medium-sized pears
125ml (4fl oz) water
½ tsp grated fresh ginger root
2 cloves
1 cardamom pod, split open slightly to allow the flavour to escape
2 pinches sea salt

Place the dried apricots in a blender with about 60ml (2fl oz) water and blend to a paste. Set aside.

Quarter and core the pears then chop them into 1cm (⅓ in) pieces.

Put the apricot paste and chopped pears in a saucepan with the remaining ingredients and cook over a medium heat for 15 minutes until soft.

Apple Sauce *(Serves 4)*

6 eating apples, preferably organic
250ml (9fl oz) unsweetened apple juice
¼ tsp ground cinnamon

Chop the apples into 2cm (¾ in) cubes, cutting out the core.

Put the apple juice in a pan and bring it to the boil. Once boiling, add the cinnamon and apples immediately.

Reduce the heat and simmer for about 20 minutes or until the apple is soft. Serve hot or cold.

Baked Apples *(Serves 4)*

This recipe can also be made using pears.

> 4 eating apples, preferably organic
> 75g (2½ oz) raisins
> 1 tbsp ground cinnamon
> ¼ tsp grated nutmeg or ground cardamom
> 30g (1oz) sunflower seeds
> ¼ tsp organic lemon peel or 1 tsp lemon juice
> 500ml (18fl oz) unsweetened apple juice
> Ghee or unsalted butter (optional)

Preheat the oven to 180°C/350°F/Gas mark 4.

Core the apples and place them in a deep baking dish.

Mix the raisins, spices, seeds and lemon peel together and stuff the mixture firmly into the cored apples.

Pour the apple juice into the dish and, if you wish, dot a little knob of ghee or butter on top of each apple. Cover and bake for 45 minutes or until tender.

Debbie's Fruit Crumble *(Serves 4)*

Most people won't realize this is a guilt-free dessert!

> 2 large cooking apples, peeled, cored and sliced
> 115g (4oz) raspberries or any other seasonal soft fruit (frozen forest fruits are good too)
> 3 tbsp water
> 4 tbsp maple syrup
> 85g (3oz) ground almonds
> 30g (1oz) walnut pieces
> 85g (3oz) coarse porridge oats

55g (2oz) wheat-free plain flour
85g (3oz) butter or soya spread

Preheat the oven to 200°C/400°F/Gas mark 6.

Put the fruit, water and 2 tablespoons of the maple syrup in a baking dish, stirring a little to mix in the syrup. Cover and place in the oven to soften the fruit whilst you make the crumble (don't leave it too long though).

Put all the remaining ingredients into a bowl and mix together thoroughly – you should aim to make lots of little crumbs. Sprinkle the mixture evenly over the fruit.

Bake for 20–25 minutes until the topping is slightly browned and the fruit juices are bubbling up from beneath.

Apricot Fool *(Makes 4 generous portions)*

This is a great dessert that is also equally nice for breakfast.

225g (8oz) organic Hunza apricots, soaked overnight
Juice and rind of 1 lemon
3 tbsp maple syrup
285ml (½ pint) natural yogurt (try to use Greek-style sheep's yogurt instead of cow's)

Simmer the apricots in a little water to soften.

Drain off any excess fluid and then liquidize the apricots until you have a thick purée.

Add all the other ingredients and then liquidize again.

Pour the mixture into serving dishes and refrigerate until you are ready to serve.

Baking

Soda Bread *(Makes 1 large loaf)*

This bread is best eaten within 24 hours of baking. For a nice variation to this recipe, add chopped rosemary or thyme to the dough.

> 455g (1lb) wheat-free flour
> 6 heaped tsp wheat-free baking powder
> ½ tsp salt
> 4 heaped tbsp natural yogurt
> About 300ml (10fl oz) warm water

Preheat the oven to 200°C/400°F/Gas mark 6.

Sift the flour into a large bowl. Add the baking powder and salt and mix well with a spoon.

Now add the yogurt and enough water to form a dough. Place the dough on a non-stick baking sheet and spread it out a little. Bake in the centre of the oven for about 45 minutes until firm and golden on the top. Leave it to cool on the baking sheet.

Maple Syrup Cookies *(Makes about 10 cookies)*

> 55g (2oz) oatmeal flour
> 55g (2oz) wheat-free plain flour
> 2 tbsp walnut pieces or almonds
> 3 tbsp maple syrup
> ¼ tsp baking powder
> 2 tbsp mild organic olive oil (or blended olive and sunflower oil)
> 1–2 tbsp tepid water, according to consistency

Preheat the oven to 150°C/300°F/Gas mark 2.

Place the flours, nuts, maple syrup, baking powder and oil in a bowl and blend it well using your hands. As with all wheat-free doughs, the mix tends to need a little more time to absorb the fluids so, once it is all mixed, it's a good idea to let the dough rest. Mould into walnut-shell sized balls – if it seems too dry to do this, add the water gradually until the shape holds.

Place the balls on a lined baking tray and flatten them slightly.

Bake for 20 minutes until evenly cooked. The maple syrup tends not to darken deeply but will impart a gentle sweetness to the cookie.

Fruity Muffins *(Makes 12 muffins)*

> 170g (6oz) wheat-free plain flour
> 115g (4oz) polenta (fine cornmeal)
> 1 tbsp baking powder
> 3 tbsp maple syrup
> 2 tbsp mild organic olive oil (or blended olive and sunflower oil)
> 180ml (6fl oz) almond, soya or rice milk
> 140ml (5fl oz) unsweetened apple juice
> 225g (8oz) berries, fresh or frozen – any type

Preheat the oven to 200°C/400°F/Gas mark 6.

Sift the flour, polenta and baking powder into a bowl.

Mix the maple syrup, oil, milk and apple juice together in a bowl or jug. Add the liquid to the dry ingredients and mix to produce a runny batter.

Now add the fruit to the batter and give it a quick stir.

Divide the mixture between the cups of a 12-hole bun tray. Bake for 15 minutes or until golden and the muffins are just shrinking from the sides.

Snacks

Dry Roasted Pumpkin Seeds *(Makes about 1 cup)*

> 115g (4oz) raw pumpkin seeds
> 1 tsp ground coriander
> ½ tsp ground cumin
> ½ tsp rock or sea salt
> ¼ tsp turmeric

Mix all the ingredients together, place in a large saucepan and cook over a low heat until the pumpkin seeds begin to pop – about 10 minutes.

Stir and cook for a further 1–2 minutes. Cool before eating.

Scrummy Sunflower Seeds *(Makes about 2 cups)*

Sunflower seeds are great for nibbling or as a garnish for main dishes – they're also rich in potassium and zinc.

> 225g (8oz) fresh sunflower seeds

Warm a non-stick saucepan over a low heat. After 2 minutes, add the sunflower seeds.

Toast for 15–20 minutes, stirring occasionally. Cool before eating.

Turmeric Top-up

Mix ¼ teaspoon of turmeric powder with a little honey and eat this twice a day. It helps when all the muscles, ligaments and joints feel tender and fluid-logged. It is also a good remedy for acute and chronic coughs.

Beverages

Ginger Tea *(Serves 1)*

This tea eases morning sickness and is gently detoxifying.

> 2.5cm (1in) piece of fresh ginger root, cut into thin slices
> 1 litre (1¾ pints) water

Simmer the ginger slices in the water for 20 minutes. Strain and drink a mug of this tea as your first drink of the day. Drink the rest at 3–4 hourly intervals.

If you wish you could sweeten it with ½ a teaspoon of honey – but remember your total quota of honey during the day is only 2 teaspoons and it should only be added when the drink has cooled down a bit.

Tea to aid Digestion *(Serves 2)*

This can be drunk after any meal – it is a *very* good digestive aid.

> 500ml (18fl oz) water
> 1 tsp fennel seeds
> 1 tsp cumin seeds
> 1 tsp coriander seeds

Bring the water to the boil. Put all the seeds in a blender and pour in the boiling water. Grind the seeds with the water, strain and serve.

Chamomile Tea *(Serves 1)*

This tea is soothing on the nerves and good before bedtime. It can also calm the digestion, however it should not be drunk regularly.

250ml (9fl oz) water
1 tbsp dried chamomile

Bring the water to boil in a saucepan. Add the chamomile, turn off the heat and let it sit for 30 minutes. Strain and serve.

Lemongrass and Nettle Tea *(Serves 1)*

This is a good tonic for the kidneys and is especially good for kapha and pitta.

340ml (12fl oz) water
1 tbsp lemongrass
1 tsp chopped nettles

Bring the water to the boil in a saucepan. Add the lemongrass and nettles. Cover the saucepan, turn the heat to low and simmer gently for 5 minutes.

Now turn the heat off and let it sit for another 20 minutes. Strain and serve hot or cold.

Peppermint Tea *(Serves 1)*

This is good for the nerves and heart palpitations caused by nerve imbalances. It also aids weak digestion. Peppermint counteracts homoeopathic remedies so avoid it if you are on homoeopathic medication.

250ml (9fl oz) water
1 tsp fresh peppermint leaves or 2 tsp dried

Bring the water to the boil in a saucepan. Add the peppermint, cover the saucepan and turn off the heat. Let it sit for 15 minutes or more.

Strain and serve.

Hot Milk with Nutmeg *(Serves 1)*

This is very good for calming nerves and relieving insomnia. It shouldn't be drunk too often by kapha mothers.

250ml (9fl oz) goat's milk or rice milk
½ tsp ground nutmeg

Bring milk to the boil, reduce heat and stir in the nutmeg. Simmer for 5 minutes, allow to cool a little and then serve.

Water

'What do I need a recipe for water for?' I hear you ask. Well, I'm only kidding – it isn't a recipe, just a reminder to drink lots of water. You can drink up to 3 litres of water every day, at perhaps a glass every hour, at room temperature or warmer. It helps to keep you hydrated and healthy, as well as being a good detox by itself.

Avoid ice in your water (in fact avoid all iced drinks) – the chill of the ice shocks your pancreas into sluggishness. Your pancreas is vital to digestion. Many muscle and joint problems are caused by food that has been inadequately digested due to pancreatic dysfunction.

Appendix B

Letters from Gentle Birth Mothers

This is just a small selection of the many letters I have received over the years.

Mary, Steve and Gemma – January 1999

Dear Gowri,

Like air traffic control, you helped us to land safely and we birthed at home in water with no pain relief needed. You guided us home.

Forever thankful

Louise, midwife – January 2000

Dear Gowri,

You gave me the strength and positivity to deliver my daughter, Isabella, gently and peacefully into the world. I strongly believe that the treatments and care you and your team gave helped transform fears about my own capabilities and made me focus on a positive outcome. I had a five-hour labour, without analgesia, and delivered Isabella, who weighed 6lbs 12oz, in water, without tearing. It has been one of the most amazing experiences of my life.

I felt so nurtured and cherished from the beginning of my pregnancy, which led to a great sense of peace and well-being for both me and the baby. I can't thank you enough for your amazing abilities to bring a new awareness to birth, especially when our society is so geared up to hi-tech care and monitoring. You are an inspiration.

Gabby – August 2001

As expected, Maisy arrived a week late, but when she came, she rushed quickly into the world. Contractions were text book and we trotted off to hospital, only to be disappointingly told that I was only 1cm dilated and would probably not deliver the baby until the following evening.

So I hooked myself up to your tape on my Walkman and sat in the bath. Three hours later, I was fully dilated and ready to push. My waters broke at 12.30pm and Maisy arrived at 3.30pm. Paul would say that my weekly reflexology and Creative Healing treatments made me a nicer, heavily pregnant person to live with, and we both agree that it made Maisy's birth exciting and reasonably enjoyable and quick.

Thank you for all your advice. I was surprised at my own body, and felt empowered by the whole experience.

Nicky

Gowri, you inspired my confidence because you have all-round ability and insight. You have crossed the divide between the conventional and the alternative, which made me feel very secure.

Phillipa – August 2000

My pre-labour was long. It started at 3 a.m. on Friday morning and then I went into full labour at 3 p.m. on Saturday afternoon. My contractions were painful early on, leaving me unable to sleep, so my big obstacle was not tiring too early.

The birth unit was empty except for one other mother, so my partner and I were able to move around and change our scenery. I used a TENS machine and then was in water for a long time.

The reason I got through it and found it such a positive experience is due to the self-hypnosis and visualization techniques you taught me. All along, I recalled my safe place and used my breath constantly. I was conscious of everything but felt nothing could touch me or harm me.

Your programme teaches every mother to reclaim a positive attitude towards birth, which is fast disappearing in this age of medical intervention. My baby is very lucky to have had such a good start and journey into the world.

Lara – December 2002

I was so terrified of the whole ordeal, but you made me feel invincible. Great teamwork between John, you and myself enabled me to escape to my safe place throughout the pain.

Diana Dixon – January 2000

Of all my antenatal classes, I most looked forward to Gowri's self-hypnosis session for its relentless positivity. Each week, I'd hear about manageable, joyful labour and a body fully capable of delivering a baby. During the actual labour, I often thought of Gowri's 'jelly' image and took my mind to its safe place. And I always concentrated on maximum relaxation between contractions. The supplementary yoga and (very reasonable) dietary advice also contributed to a highly-successful, pain-relief-free, efficient – and even pleasurable, in its own way – labour and delivery.

Donna Air – September 2003

Dear Gowri

I wanted to say a huge thank you for your care and patience, making my birthing experience as amazing as it was. It was a day that I will never forget! Thank you for helping my daughter arrive safe and sound. Damian and I are both extremely grateful and are big fans of your wonderful work.

Heather Parker – September 2003

Dear Gowri, Debbie and Kasia

Just a note to thank you so much for your unbelievable support, strength and guidance throughout my pregnancy and the birth of our precious son Levi. It was by far the most amazing and best day of our lives. Jake and I are both so happy that you were there. I know the experience would have been very different without you and not nearly as positive and rewarding.

Gowri Motha is 'the most special obstetrician working in this country now'. Taken from the article 'The Experts' Expert' (*Observer* magazine, 1990) by Michel Odent, obstetrician and pioneer of waterbirths.

Appendix C

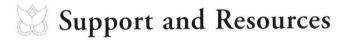

Support and Resources

Contacting Dr Gowri Motha

Dr Motha and her team work at two venues in London. If you would like to enrol on the Gentle Birth Method programme at these venues please contact them directly:

Viveka Clinic
27a Queen's Terrace
St John's Wood
London
NW8 6EA
Tel: 020 7483 3788

The Jeyarani Centre
South Woodford
London
E18 2AL
Tel: 020 8530 1146
www.gentlebirthmethod.com
E-mail: gowrimotha@jeyarani.com

Referrals
Most clients are self-referred by personal recommendation through friends. Mothers enrolled on to the birth unit at St John and St Elizabeth's Hospital at St John's Wood, London NW8 have easy access to Dr Motha's clinic at Viveka.

NHS connection
The Jeyarani Way Gentle Birth Method will become available within the NHS at Queen Charlotte's and Chelsea Hospital, East Acton, West London, as part of a research study into integrating complementary and conventional care in obstetrics. The project is due to commence in 2004.

Self-hypnosis and Visualization Classes
Classes are held on Mondays at 6.30 p.m. at the Viveka clinic. Mothers and their partners can enrol onto a course of 4 initial classes, each of 90 minutes' duration. Couples are encouraged to attend top-up classes. Classes are also held at:
Lotus Lifestyle Yoga Centre, Chelsea Design Centre, Chelsea Harbour, London SW10 0XE. (Telephone to book courses at this venue: 020 7349 9991. Website: www.lotuslifestyle.com)

For classes at other times and venues, please look up our website for details.

Dr Motha works with a team of practitioners who have been trained by her and work with her. They also work independently:
Kasia Ayub – Jeyarani Gentle Birth Practitioner, Reflexologist, Creative healer, Bowen therapist and Reiki healer.
Tel: 077485 90645

Debbie Linger – Jeyarani Gentle Birth Practitioner, teaches the Jeyarani Way Self-hypnosis and visualization programme for birth preparation, Hypnotherapist, Reflexologist, Creative healer, Bowen therapist and Reiki healer.
Tel: 020 8989 1200

Sherine Lovegrove – Jeyarani Gentle Birth Practitioner, teaches the Jeyarani Way Self-hypnosis and visualization programme for birth preparation, Psychotherapist, Hypnotherapist, Reflexologist, Creative healer, Reiki healer and Midwife.
Tel: 020 8444 2249

Marion McKay – Jeyarani Gentle Birth Practitioner, Reflexologist, Creative healer, Bowen therapist, Reiki healer.
Tel: 020 8558 8343

Leslie Wrenn-Brown – Creative healer and Reiki healer.
Tel: 07986 030883

Jeyarani Associates that have set up their own practices

United Kingdom

Judith Davies SRN – Creative healer, Reflexologist, Nurse, Midwife and Jeyarani Gentle Birth Practitioner.
Address: 1, Vine House, Eardisley, Herefordshire HR3 6NJ.
Tel: 01544 327022

Heather Guerrini – Reflexologist, Creative healer, Nurse, NCT birth educator, Jeyarani Gentle Birth Practitioner.
Based in West London.
Tel: 020 7352 0245

Rachel Foux – Creative healer, Reflexologist, Counsellor, Jeyarani Gentle Birth Practitioner (teaches the Jeyarani Way Self-hypnosis and visualization classes).
Based in Kings Langley, Hertfordshire.
Tel: 01923 270027

Viola Martens – Creative healer, Reflexologist and Jeyarani Gentle Birth Practitioner.
Based in Southgate, London N14.
Tel: 020 8368 4789

Helen Dennis – Creative healer, Reflexologist, Reiki healer and Jeyarani Gentle Birth Practitioner.
Based in East Ham, London.
Tel: 020 8471 9118

Debbie Pumfrett – Creative healer and Reiki healer
Based in Hertfordshire.
E-mail: debbiepumfrett@dial.pipex.com

Brian Beber and Bea Kirsopp – Creative healers, Reflexologists. Brian is also a Homoeopath, psychotherapist, podiatrist and physiotherapist – wow!
Address: Crown Treatment Centre, 2 Crown Lane, Littleport, Cambridgeshire CB6 1PP.
Tel: 01353 863218
www.hteam.addr.com

Antonella Ravera – Reflexologist, Creative healer, Shiatsu practitioner, yoga teacher, Jeyarani Gentle Birth Practitioner.
Based in Norwich.
Tel: 01603 464517
E-mail: anton.ravera@ntlworld.com

Japan

Chika Nagasu – Reflexologist and Jeyarani Gentle Birth Practitioner.
Based in Fujisawa City, Kanagawa, Japan.
E-mail: m-nagasu@oecf.go.jp

India

Dr Sister Angelina MS, Creative healer, Reflexologist, Jeyarani Gentle Birth Practitioner and General Surgeon.
Based at St John's Medical College, Bangalore, India.
E-mail: vtmj@vsnl.net

Recommended Dietary Supplements
Important supplements, recommended to mothers during pregnancy:
Pre-natal or pregnancy vitamins. Recommended brands Biocare or Solgar.
Probiotics. Recommended brands Biocare or Dr Udo.
Herbal teas for pregnancy – Jeyarani
Baladi Choornam – Jeyarani
Dhanwantaram pills (baby pills) – Jeyarani
Homeopathic Tissue Salt Programme – Jeyarani
Essential fatty acids – omega 3 (also omega 6 and 9). For those who would like to use fish oils I recommend a blend called MorDHA. In general and for vegetarians I recommend flaxseed and hemp seed oils. (Reputable brands include: Mother Hemp Oil and Dr Udo's oils.)

Optional:
Digestive enzymes. Recommended brands Biocare (Digest Aid), or Dr Udo's.
Essential sugars Ambrotose – by Mannatech.
Vitamin A or Beta-carotene. Recommended brands Centrum, Biocare or Solgar. (Caution: Vitamin A should be taken with care during pregnancy take no more that 2000–5000 IU per day of Vitamin A. Beta–Carotene (8000 IU per day) is a safer alternative to Vitamin A as the body does not store Beta-carotene, but the body can convert this to Vitamin A as required.)

Suppliers:
Health food shops usually have the Biocare, Solgar and Dr Udo's ranges, or they can order them for you. They also sell Bach Flower Remedies and essential oils for aromatherapy.

Large supermarkets usually have the Centrum range.

The Jeyarani Centre sells Ambrotose (tel: 020 8530 1146).

The Nutri Centre: www.nutricentre.co.uk; tel: 020 7436 5122. (Sells Biocare, Solgar, Dr Udo's products MorDHA and other helpful oils; Homoeopathic remedies; Bach Flower Remedies; essential oils for aromatherapy; Ayurvedic products.)

Planet Organic does mail order: 42 Westbourne Grove, London W2 5SH; tel: 020 7727 2227. (Sells same products as The Nutri Centre, listed above.)

The Health Store: http://www.healthstoreuk.com (Sells the Solgar and Dr Udo brands.)

G. Baldwin and Co.: www.baldwins.co.uk; tel: 020 7703 5550. (Sells herbs for Herbal Tea and Bach Flower Remedies.)

Recommended Ayurvedic product supplier

Ayurvedic suppliers: www.tattvaayurveda.com. (For Triphala powder and oil, medicinal turmeric, sesame oil and coconut oil for self-massage, Vitex Nirgundi tincture.)

Recommended Homoeopathic product suppliers

Ainsworth Homoeopathic Pharmacy: www.ainsworth.com

Helios Homoeopathic Pharmacy: www.helios.co.uk; tel: 01892 536393

Weleda (UK) Ltd: www.weleda.co.uk; tel: 0115 944 8200

The Nutri Centre: www.nutricentre.co.uk; tel: 020 7436 5122

The Jeyarani Way Gentle Birth Method Products

All of the following products are available on request:

From the Jeyarani website: www.gentlebirthmethod.com

By post: The Jeyarani Centre, 34 Cleveland Road, South Woodford, London, E18 2AL

By phone: 020 8530 1146

Herbs and Nutritional supplements

Herbal tea

Baladi Choornam Herbs (to make the drink)
Dhanwantaram pills (baby pills)
Homeopathic Tissue Salt Programme – for each month of pregnancy
Homeopathic Labour Kit (containing the common remedies that you may need during labour, including Rescue Remedy – Bach Flower)
Ambrotose (essential sugars)

Jeyarani Oils
Ayurvedic herbal Pregnancy and Anti-stretch mark oil (150ml)
Aromatherapy Pregnancy and Anti-stretch mark oil (some mothers may prefer this as it has floral essences and is lighter than the Ayurvedic oil)
Perineal and Vaginal oil (Internal Birthing Oil) (an Ayurvedic formula, well researched, helps to prevent tearing and protect your perineum)
Jeyarani Aromatherapy Labour Massage Oil (can be used with the recommended Creative Healing massage techniques during labour)

Jeyarani Guides
Dietary Advice and Recipes for Pregnant Mothers. (This booklet contains all the recipes found in this book and more.)

Self-hypnosis and Visualization tapes and CDs
'The Jeyarani Way': Prepare for a Natural Birth with Self-hypnosis and Visualisation by Dr Gowri Motha. (Contents: Self-hypnosis, visualization and birth rehearsal.) Audio tape and CD
Gentle Birthing 'The Jeyarani Way' Labour Tape by Dr Gowri Motha. (To listen to throughout labour.) Audio tape and CD
The Jeyarani Way – Turning a Breech Baby by Dr Gowri Motha. (Deep relaxations and visualizations to help turn a breech presentation.) CD only
The Twin Tape by Dr Gowri Motha. (Helping mothers who are pregnant with twins to prepare for a natural birth with Self-hypnosis and visualization.) Audio tape and CD
Toning Up After Birth 'The Jeyarani Way' by Dr Gowri Motha. (Post-natal visualization and deep relaxation to help you regain your pre-pregnant shape,

size and tone, and be more beautiful than ever before!) Audio tape and CD

The Sleep Tape by Dr Gowri Motha. (A general relaxation tape with specific mind–body conditioning suggestions to induce deep restful sleep. Can help you to quickly go back to sleep.) CD only

Jeyarani Mantras for Meditation. (Gayatri Mantra and Om Nama Shivaya Mantra) By Dr Gowri Motha (For use during yoga, meditation, chanting and can help you to relax and become more spiritual. Also good as background music to your therapies.) CD only.

Videos and DVDs

How to Prepare for a Safe and Easy Waterbirth, presented by Dr Gowri Motha. (Shows some actual waterbirths.) Available in video and DVD format.

Creative Healing Massage Demonstration for Birth Preparation (for home use), presented by Dr Gowri Motha. (Shows all the Creative healing techniques that can be performed on the pregnant mother at home, both in pregnancy and labour.) Available in DVD format.

Jeyarani Yoga for Pregnancy. (20–30-minute basic yoga routine for use during pregnancy. Recommended for daily use to achieve birthfitness. Also shows the 'funny walks'.) Available in DVD format

Miscellaneous

Jeyarani Pregnancy Candle (An aromatherapy candle to be used during your Self-hypnosis sessions and your Creative Healing massage treatments. Has a light floral fragrance.)

Post-natal waist trimming support panty. To be worn every day for a month after giving birth. Recommended in Creative Healing to regain your waist and tummy contours very quickly after birth.

The Jeyarani Way, Gentle Birth Method Package – from A–Z

A comprehensive package of Jeyarani products for pregnancy, the package includes:

Herbal tea (5 months' supply)

Baladi Choornam Herbs (to make the drink) (5 months' supply)

Dhanwantaram pills (baby pills) (5 months' supply)

Homoeopathic Tissue Salt Programme – for each month of pregnancy

Homoeopathic Labour Kit (containing the common remedies that you may need during labour)

Ayurvedic herbal Pregnancy and Anti-stretch mark oil (300ml)

Perineal and Vaginal oil (an Ayurvedic formula, well researched, helps to prevent tearing and protect your perineum)

'The Jeyarani Way': Prepare for a natural birth with Self-hypnosis and Visualization, by Dr Gowri Motha. (Contents: Self-hypnosis, visualization and birth rehearsal.) Audio tape and CD (please indicate which one you prefer)

Gentle Birthing 'The Jeyarani Way' Labour Tape, by Dr Gowri Motha. (To listen to throughout labour.) Audio tape

Toning Up after Birth 'The Jeyarani Way', by Dr Gowri Motha. (Post-natal visualization and deep relaxation to help you regain your pre-pregnant shape, size and tone, and be more beautiful than ever before!) Audio tape and CD (please indicate which one you prefer)

How to Prepare for a Safe and Easy Waterbirth, presented by Dr Gowri Motha. (Shows some actual waterbirths.) Available in video and DVD format (please indicate which one you prefer)

Creative Healing Massage Demonstration for Birth Preparation (for home use), presented by Dr Gowri Motha. (Shows all the Creative healing techniques that can be performed on the pregnant mother at home, both in pregnancy and labour.) Available in DVD format

Jeyarani Yoga for Pregnancy. (20–30-minute basic yoga routine for use during pregnancy. Recommended for daily use to achieve birthfitness. Also shows the 'funny walks'.) Available in DVD format

The Therapist Pack

This pack is put together for therapists who are not Jeyarani Gentle Birth Practitioners, but do complementary therapies and wish to help the pregnant mother follow The Jeyarani Way Gentle Birth Method.

The therapist pack includes:

Creative Healing Massage Demonstration for Birth Preparation (for home use), presented by Dr Gowri Motha. (Shows all the Creative healing techniques that can be performed on the pregnant mother at home, both in pregnancy and labour.) Available in DVD format.

Creative Healing, Special Applications DVD. (Includes additional treatments that may be useful when treating the pregnant mother, i.e. pancreatic treatment, liver drainage, heart treatment.)

Information on courses that the therapist might like to take, e.g. Creative Healing and Bowen therapy.

A brief guide on Reflexology during pregnancy.

Information on Jeyarani herbs and oils.

Other Useful Contact Details:
Creative Healing Associates and Schools
Patricia and John Bradley. Founders of the Joseph B. Stephenson's Creative Healing Foundation, 66 Sequoia Circle, Santa Rosa, CA. 95401, USA.

Rebecca (Becky) Jackson. Principal of the Northwest Arkansas School of Massage, USA. Teacher of Creative Healing. P.O. Box 107, Combs, AR, 72721, USA; tel: 00-1-479-677-2671

Louise Hunt, 264 Coronado, Long Beach, CA, 90803, USA.

Katharina Krogbäumker
Based in Germany.
Tel: 00 49 (0) 2581 782299
E-mail: BeaMaKarina@aol.com
www.sanftewege.de

Simone Moter
Based in Germany
Tel: 09642 1183488
E-mail: simone@moter.de

Katerina Papkonstanstinou
Based in Greece
E-mail: gconcept@otenet.gr

Reflexology Associates and Associations
Association of Reflexologists, 27 Old Gloucester Street, London WC1N 3XX;
tel/fax: 01892 512 612, www.reflexology.org.

Hazel Goodwin, former Chairperson of the Association of Reflexologists. Based in West Sussex.

Jennie Levick. National Director, International Institute of Reflexology, 146 Upperthorpe, Walkley, Sheffield, South Yorkshire S6 3NF. Tel: 01142 812100. www.reflexology-uk.net

Renee Tanner. International Federation of Reflexologists. Tel: 020 8686 4781

Kristine Walker. School of Reflexology, 223 Hartington Road, Brighton, East Sussex BN2 3PA

Bowen Therapist Associates and School
Bowen School and Bowen Foundation, Enterprise House, 113–115 George Lane, London E18 1AB; tel: 020 8556 7586. Susanna Hall, Bowen practitioner and tutor.

Fiona Meeks. Bowen practitioner, Reflexologist and former Midwife.
Based in East Sheen, London.
Tel: 020 8876 3010.

Cranio-sacral Associates and School
Thomas Attlee, Principal of the College of Cranio-sacral Therapy, 9 St George Mews, Primrose Hill, London NW1 8XE; tel: 020 7586 0120

Yoga Associates

Francoise Freedman. Founder of Birthlight Yoga. Author of several books and videos on yoga. Based in Cambridge, UK.
www.birthlight.com

Nell Lindsell. Founder of Yogabugs. Specializes in pregnancy yoga and yoga for children.
www.yogabugs.com

Kate Appleton. Teaches general, pregnancy and post-natal yoga.
E-mail: katy@appleyoga.com
www.appleyoga.com

Lotus Lifestyle Yoga Centre. Offers pregnancy yoga, children's yoga and The Jeyarani Way Gentle Birth self-hypnosis and visualization courses.
Address: 3rd Floor, The Design Centre, Chelsea Harbour, London SW10 0XE.
Tel: 020 7349 9991
www.lotuslifestyle.com

Ayurvedic Associates and College

Dr Palitha Serasinghe. Assistant Director and Principal Lecturer at The College of Ayurveda (UK), 20 Annes Grove, Great Linford, Milton Keynes, NK14 5DR. (Courses are held in London.)
E-mail: Palitha.Serasinghe@ntlworld.com
www.ayurvedacollege.co.uk

Zia Rawji. Ayurvedic Counsellor and Reflexologist. Based in Taplow, Bucks.
Tel: 01628 660655

Waterbirth

Splashdown Water Birth Services Ltd, 17 Wellington Terrace, Harrow on the Hill, Middlesex HA1 3EP; tel: 0870 4444403. www.waterbirth.co.uk

Cookie and Michael Harkin. Babyswim Australia, 23 Fuschia Street, Blackburn, Victoria 3130, Australia

Lucy Ann De-Vletter. Aqua Baby Birthpool Hire, De Genestetraat 27, 4873 CP Etten-leur, Nederlands. www.aquababy.nl

Institute of Complementary Medicine
P.O. Box 194, London SE16 1QZ; tel: 020 7237 5165
(For details of local complementary therapy practitioners, send an addressed envelope and two loose stamps)

Homeopathic Medical Association
6 Livingstone Road, Gravesend, Kent DA12 5AZ; tel: 01474 560336.
www.homeopathy.org

Further reading:
Birth and Beyond, by Dr Yehudi Gordon. Published by Vermilion, London, 2002. ISBN: 0-09-185694-9

Birth without Violence by Frederick Leboyer. Published by Mandarin, 1991. ISBN: 0-7493-0642-4

Primal Health: Understanding the Critical Period Between Conception and the First Birthday by Michel Odent. Published by Clairview Books, 2002. ISBN: 1902636333

Birth Reborn by Michel Odent. Published by Random House, 1986. ISBN: 0394712986

The Caesarean by Michel Odent. Published by Free Association Books, 2004. ISBN: 1853437182

Homoeopathy for Pregnancy, Birth and Your Baby's First Year by Miranda Castro. Published by St Martin's Griffin, 1993. ISBN: 0-312-08809-4

Homoeopathy for Midwives (and All Pregnant Women) by Peter Webb. Published by British Homoeopathic Association, 1992. ISBN: 094671701X

Craniosacral Therapy by John E. Upledger and Jon D. Vredevoogd. Published by Eastland Press, 1983. ISBN: 0-939616-01-7

Perfect Health by Deepak Chopra. Published by Bantam, 2001. ISBN: 0553813676

Make
www.thorsonselement.com
your online sanctuary

Get online information, inspiration and guidance to help you on the path to physical and spiritual well-being. Drawing on the integrity and vision of our authors and titles, and with health advice, articles, astrology, tarot, a meditation zone, author interviews and events listings, www.thorsonselement.com is a great alternative to help create space and peace in our lives.

So if you've always wondered about practising yoga, following an allergy-free diet, using the tarot or getting a life coach, we can point you in the right direction.

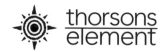

thorsons
element